Raising Chase – A Fight For Life

©2025 Donna Kirk

Raising Chase – the moments of darkness

When its dark and the world seems a little off kilter, I take a few moments to focus on breathing. In and out. In and out. I strain to see if for just once, I hear those hidden rosy bellows called lungs fill with the life-giving oxygen that allows me to live. I work hard to imagine what it must feel like for my son to for just one moment not labour for breath. To grasp his frustration and glimpse even an iota of the physical and mental anguish his body is forced to endure.

For 23 years, these dark moments have crept into my nights but rarely my days. The days leave little room for reflection, consumed instead by medical routines, physiotherapy, hospital visits, and relentless research. Even now that he has left home and lives an hour away, my thoughts often stray to his welfare despite my determination to push them aside allowing him to live his best life.

Raising Chase has been a privilege and an honour.

It has also been a challenge, a lifelong journey of learning and an adventure worthy of a book. This is our story. A mother, a son and a journey of discovery.

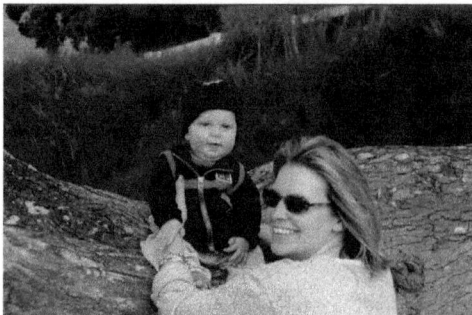

The moment had arrived. A moment I had somehow managed to avoid for exactly twelve hours and forty-six minutes since bringing Chase home. I had dodged, delayed, and even considered bribing his father to step in, but there was no escaping it now.

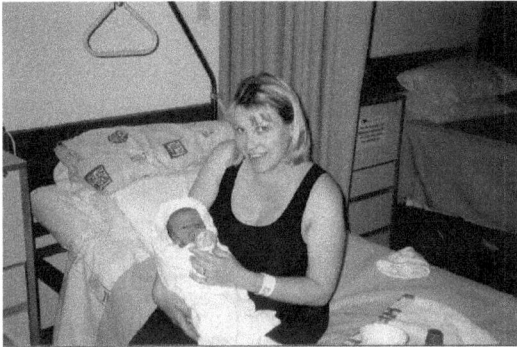

Chase needed a nappy change, and I was the only adult in the room.

Now, don't get me wrong. I had read about this. I had watched the videos. Although refusing to attend prenatal classes, I had watched a you tube video where an impossibly calm midwife demonstrated the "quick and easy" method on a plastic doll. But let me tell you, nothing – absolutely nothing – prepares you for the reality of a wriggling, wailing, and very much alive newborn with an alarmingly full nappy. And this baby was all legs and no body so it was about to get interesting.

I approached the changing table like a soldier heading into battle. Supplies? Check. Fresh nappy? Check. Wipes? Check. A slightly overinflated sense of confidence? Also, check.

I unsnapped the onesie with trembling fingers, revealing the crime scene within. The sheer scope of destruction defied logic. How could one tiny human produce something of this magnitude? Was it physics? Witchcraft? A prank?

Chase, blissfully unaware of my inner turmoil, cooed up at me, his little legs kicking dangerously close to the danger zone. "Alright, buddy," I muttered. "Let's do this."

Step one: Undo the nappy.

Easy enough. Except the moment I pulled back the tabs, Chase took this as his cue to wriggle like an eel, sending a mild panic through my veins. I attempted to fold the nappy in half, as per my online research, but instead, it folded in such a way that I ended up with an alarming amount of questionable substance on my hand.

I froze. Chase gurgled. The cat, sensing an opportunity for chaos, wandered closer, sniffing the air suspiciously.

"Don't even think about it," I warned her.

Step two: Wipes.

I reached for them with my untainted hand, only to discover that, in my preoccupation with not gagging, I had forgotten to actually open the pack. With an elbow, I tried to wrestle the plastic lid open, only to have the entire thing topple off the table and onto the floor, landing just out of reach.

Chase lay there with a look I can only describe as incredulous.

"This is funny to you?" I asked, balancing precariously as I stretched for the wipes with my foot. Success! Except now I had baby wipes stuck to my toes, which made me question every single life decision that had led me to this exact moment.

Step three: The Cleanup.

Once armed with wipes, I went in, hands shaking, desperately trying to maintain some dignity. Chase, clearly delighted by this unexpected entertainment, flailed his arms and legs, managing to kick the soiled nappy, which then flipped—yes, flipped—onto my sleeve.

The cat, now far too interested in proceedings, attempted to get a closer look.

"Nope. Out." I pointed sternly toward the door, flapping my dirty arm at her.

I somehow managed to wipe this eel of a baby down without further catastrophe, though I did have to chase a rogue wipe across the changing table like an amateur magician failing a card trick. Just as I reached the final step, something horrible happened.

Chase, in his infinite newborn wisdom, decided now was a great time to provide a fresh offering. Now at this stage in our lives we had no idea at all what was to come. All I knew was that this poop was the grossest thing I had ever experienced.

And now, it was there running down my hand.

There are no words for the sounds that came out of my mouth in that moment. None. It was part gasp, part shriek, part primal wail. The cat, alarmed by my outburst, bolted down the passage. Chase, unfazed, kicked out a leg, threw an uncoordinated arm up and for a new born had the agility of a professional wrestler.

I had two options: Lose all sense of dignity and cry, or power through. I chose the latter (though I did make a mental note to dramatically retell this story to anyone who would listen).

With all the grace of a sleep-deprived contortionist, I cleaned my hand, retrieved a fresh nappy, and attempted what I hoped would be the final step. But the thing about nappies is that they require some level of coordination, and mine was rapidly deteriorating.

"Alright, just stay still," I muttered, attempting to manoeuvre his wiggling legs into the correct position. One leg in. Okay. Second leg—

Chase kicked. The nappy flew. The cat was back at the door sniffing the air with disgust.

"NO!" I yelped, diving after it like an Olympic athlete. In my desperation, I forgot about the wipes on the floor and skidded, catching myself on the changing table just as the nappy soared past me and into the air.

Time slowed. The cat scootered like a flash and the nappy landed right in my clean hand.

There was silence.

Chase hiccupped. The cat was nowhere to be seen, clearly disgusted with the foul odour emanating from the room. I slowly removed another wad off wipes to clean myself and trying not to throw up. This wasn't to be the last time that my son would make me want to vomit.

Finally, having secured a fresh, clean nappy onto Chase, snapped his onesie closed, I stood back, victorious. I had done it. I had conquered the nappy change alone, never realising in a million years it would be this runny, this foul smelling and this gross.

Chase yawned.

And then, just as I reached for a celebratory sip of water, I heard it.

The unmistakable sound of a freshly filled nappy.

I stared at Chase. Chase stared back, completely innocent, completely adorable, and completely in need of another change.

I sighed.

The battle had been won, but the war had only just begun and what a war it would turn out to be.

The Great Baby Mix-Up (or So I Thought)

When the doctor called me back into the office, I was already sweating. Not because of the baby I was awkwardly balancing in one arm while attempting to shove a crumpled muslin cloth into my diaper bag with the other, but because I had convinced myself that I was about to star in my own personal soap opera.

Something was wrong. The doctor had sounded too serious on the phone. Too concerned. I had seen this scene in movies a hundred times—some poor unsuspecting mother, just going about her business, only to be told in a hushed voice that, due to a mix-up at the hospital, she had somehow ended up raising the wrong baby for the past four weeks.

I mean, Chase did look like me... a bit. But was that just my exhausted brain convincing me? What if I had someone else's baby? What if someone else had Chase? What if the real Chase was out there with some other family, drinking the wrong brand of formula and being wrapped in a lesser quality of muslin cloth?

Panic surged through me as I perched on the chair opposite the doctor. Chase, oblivious to my spiralling, let out a little grunt of baby satisfaction and drooled on my sleeve.

Dr. Bradley, the kind-eyed, gorgeous woman who had been our paediatrician since day one, clasped her hands together and smiled warmly. "So, I wanted to bring you in to go over some test results."

Oh, God. Here it comes.

I braced myself, gripping Chase a little tighter. "Listen, Doctor," I blurted, interrupting her before she could ruin my life with the worst news I'd ever hear. "Before you say anything, I just need to ask—how often does this sort of thing happen?"

Dr. Bradley blinked. "I—sorry, what sort of thing?"

"You know... the... mix-up."

Her brow furrowed. "Mix-up?"

I inhaled sharply. "The baby mix-up. The one where you sit me down and tell me there was some catastrophic hospital error, and this baby—my baby—actually belongs to some yoga-loving, vegan couple who probably named him 'River' or 'Zephyr' and dress him exclusively in organic hemp onesies."

Dr. Bradley stared at me, expressionless. "That... is not why I called you in."

"Oh," I exhaled. "So, no mix-up?"

"No mix-up."

I let out a nervous chuckle, waving a dismissive hand as though I hadn't just embarrassed myself beyond all recognition. "Ha! Well, that's a relief! Imagine that, huh? Me thinking I had someone else's baby. What a crazy thought! Wow. So, uh... why am I here, then?"

Dr. Bradley cleared her throat, clearly deciding to pretend the last sixty seconds had never happened. "Chase's newborn screening results came back, and we need to run some additional tests. The initial tests suggests that he has cystic fibrosis."

I nodded, waiting for my brain to catch up. "Okay. So... not a baby mix-up, but just a completely different thing."

The doctor's face softened. "I know this must be overwhelming."

Understatement of the year.

I sat there, gripping Chase, as my internal panic rebranded itself from *wrong baby* to *oh no, my actual baby has a chronic illness*. The emotional whiplash was outstanding.

Dr. Bradley began explaining what this might mean. She also explained that it wasn't definite he had it and that it wasn't that common. It was more common to be a carrier. But if he did in fact have it she reassured me that treatments had advanced, and that there was a lot of support. And all I could do was nod and pretend that my brain wasn't currently malfunctioning like an overheating laptop.

I realised I had stopped blinking. I should probably blink. And somewhere in the dark compartments of my brain a wire connected. A spark of energy threw itself into the forefront of my mind as I watched the past four weeks of runny nappies, power vomiting, lack of growth despite the constant feeding, and the skinny legs and arms all coming together into two words – Cystic Fibrosis.

Despite Dr. Bradley's reassuring words, a chilling certainty settled over me. This was it. The answer I had been unknowingly searching for, lurking in the shadows of my mind, waiting to be uncovered—whether I was ready for it or not.

Chase chose this moment to let out an impressively loud burp, startling even himself.

Dr. Bradley, without missing a beat, simply said, "That's a very healthy set of lungs."

And I, in the midst of my mental unravelling, did the only thing I could think to do.

I burst into uncontrollable laughter.

Not polite, composed laughter. No. This was deranged, high-pitched, borderline-hysterical laughter. The kind that makes strangers question if they should call someone. Chase, picking up on my vibe, joined in with his own little gurgly giggles, which only made it worse.

I gasped for breath, wiping at my eyes. "I—I thought you were going to tell me he was someone else's baby, and instead, you told me he might have cystic fibrosis. I mean—what a plot twist! Life really just keeps you on your toes, huh?"

Dr. Bradley gave me the patient, slightly weary look of a woman who had seen all kinds of maternal meltdowns in her career. "I think you might be in a little bit of shock."

"Little bit," I wheezed, trying to compose myself. "You should really lead with 'this is definitely your baby' before dropping big news. Just a suggestion."

She smiled. "I'll keep that in mind."

After a few deep breaths and a promise to set up a follow-up appointment, I walked out of that office feeling like I had just lived through a sitcom episode written by someone with a very twisted sense of humour.

Chase, my real baby—no mix-up, no Zephyr nonsense—yawned and snuggled against me. And I realised, whatever this journey looked like, this was just the beginning.

Dr. Google, M.D.

The moment the words "possible cystic fibrosis" left the doctor's lips, something primal awakened within me. My transformation was instant—I became Dr. Google, world-renowned medical researcher, working on a tight deadline.

"Don't panic," my husband, Steve, said, placing a hand on my shoulder as we walked to the car. "It's just a precautionary test."

"Totally," I said, already unlocking my phone with the speed and precision of a trained hacker.

"You know what I mean," Steve sighed. "He's perfect. He's fine."

I nodded absentmindedly, though I was already thirty-seven search results deep, speed-reading like my life depended on it. *Early symptoms. Life expectancy. Mucus?!* Oh, God. What had I just read?

Steve glanced over. "You're already Googling, aren't you?"

"Nope," I lied, tilting the screen away. "Just checking the weather."

Steve sighed again, the defeated kind of sigh that husbands of neurotic wives know all too well.

By the time we got home, I had read approximately twelve medical journals, joined two online support groups, and was fairly certain I could pass a first-year medical exam. I burst through the door like a woman on a mission, plopping Chase into his baby bouncer as I reached for my laptop.

"You know," my mother in law said from the couch, stirring her tea, "maybe don't go down the internet rabbit hole just yet."

"I am simply educating myself," I announced. "I will be responsible. Logical."

Three hours later, I was sitting on the floor surrounded by hastily scribbled notes, printouts, and a terrifyingly detailed spreadsheet categorizing every possible outcome. I had sent at least six frantic texts to my best friend, Shelly, who, unlike the rest of my overly optimistic support system, seemed to share my deeply foreboding sense of doom.

"They don't just *think* babies have CF," she texted back. "Something must've shown up. What did they say exactly?"

"Blah blah blah levels, blah blah further tests," I typed. "All I heard was *life-changing medical condition* and then the sound of my own heart exploding."

"Okay, stay calm."

"Too late," I replied. "I am one article away from becoming a full-blown pulmonologist."

Just then, Steve appeared, holding my phone. "mum wants me to tell you to step away from Google before she throws your laptop out the window."

"I CAN'T STEP AWAY, STEVE. I HAVE TO KNOW."

"Know what?"

"EVERYTHING."

Steve crouched down next to me, glancing at my notes. "Did you… create a symptom timeline?"

"Yes."

"And a—what is this? A pros and cons list of different treatments?"

"Yes."

He exhaled. "You need to calm down."

"Don't tell me to calm down, Steve. We're on a deadline!"

"The diagnosis isn't for another two weeks."

"Exactly! Time is of the essence! Do you think real doctors just sit around *waiting* for information to come to them? NO. They RESEARCH."

Steve rubbed his temples as I turned back to my laptop, ignoring his pleas for rationality. Meanwhile, my mother in law sipped her tea serenely, offering nothing but an occasional "Mm-hmm" whenever I attempted to drag her into my hysteria.

Shelly, however, was right there with me.

"Gut feeling?" she texted.

"Big gut feeling."

"Me too."

I looked over at Chase, happily gurgling in his bouncer, completely oblivious to the chaos his mother was unleashing on the internet. Steve shook his head and plopped onto the couch, resigned to my madness.

The rest of the world may have been busy reassuring me that everything was fine, but I knew better. Shelly knew better.

And Dr. Google and I had a lot more work to do.

The Battle of Emergency Room for the very first time.

Hospitals smell weird. Not necessarily bad, just... weird. A mix of industrial-strength sanitiser and mystery sadness. But I didn't have time to dwell on that. I was on a mission.

Chase, my tiny four-week-old, let out a feeble cough from his car seat, and my heart clenched. The doctors had said "possible cystic fibrosis" last week, and while we were still waiting for the final test results, my motherly instincts had already gone full *DEFCON 1*. Every wheeze, every sniffle, every slight shift in breathing had me spiralling into worst-case-scenario mode.

So here we were—me, Steve, and our probably-but-maybe-not chronically ill newborn—marching through the emergency room doors like the cast of a very underprepared medical drama.

A nurse at the front desk glanced up. "What's the reason for your visit?"

I stepped forward, gripping Chase's car seat like a woman on the edge. "He has a cough."

She gave a polite but unimpressed nod. "How long has he had it?"

"Thirty-six minutes," I said with the kind of urgency normally reserved for bomb defusals.

Steve groaned. "It's been more than that. On and off all morning."

"Which is basically a lifetime for a newborn," I snapped. "Especially *our* newborn."

The nurse looked between us. "Any fever?"

"No," Steve answered, at the same time I yelled, "*Not yet!*"

Her expression didn't change. "Alright. We'll check you in. Have a seat."

Steve and I plopped down in the waiting area, surrounded by a mix of sprained ankles, flu-ridden teenagers, and one guy who looked suspiciously like he had superglued his own hand to his ear. Chase snoozed peacefully, as if his mother *hadn't* just started an emotional campaign for urgent care.

After an eternity (which the clock insisted was only 45 minutes), we were finally called back.

Dr. Stone, a middle-aged man with glasses and the kind of hair that suggested he hadn't planned on working today, barely glanced at Chase before launching into what I suspected was his *standard new-parent reassurance speech.*

"Babies cough sometimes," he said, waving his hand as if this was supposed to make me feel better. "It's how they clear their airways. Have you been using a humidifier?"

I blinked. "A what?"

"Humidifier. It helps keep their nasal passages from drying out."

"We don't need a humidifier," I said, gripping Chase tighter. "We need *answers.*"

Steve, sensing my rising mum-rage, jumped in. "It's just that, well... he might have cystic fibrosis."

Dr. Stone nodded, still typing something on his computer. "Might. But he hasn't been diagnosed yet?"

I narrowed my eyes. "Not officially. But I know. I *know* something's not right."

Dr. Stone sighed. "Well, even if he does, a minor cough isn't necessarily alarming. Have you been suctioning his nose?"

"Excuse me?"

"With one of those little bulb syringes?"

I blinked again. "I am *not* qualified to suction things out of a human being."

He smiled in a way that made me want to throw my diaper bag at him. "It's very simple. We can show you."

"No offense, doctor, but I don't need a demonstration on booger extraction. What I *do* need is for someone to check his oxygen levels and tell me if my baby is actually okay."

He sighed, clearly debating whether it was worth arguing with a sleep-deprived, emotionally volatile mother.

Steve gave me a look that said, *Just let the man do his job.* But I wasn't having it. I had been a mother for precisely one month, and I had already learned one thing: *nobody* advocates for your baby like you do.

So, in the most aggressive yet polite way possible, I sat up straighter, cleared my throat, and channelled my inner CEO.

"With all due respect, Dr. Stone, I have been in this job for thirty days. *Thirty.* And in those thirty days, I have gained a doctorate in Baby Breathing Analysis, a master's in Fever Paranoia, and an honorary degree in Newborn Bowel Movements. If *you* had thirty days of sleep deprivation and a tiny human you were solely responsible for keeping alive, you, too, would be in full freak-out mode right now. So, please. Check his lungs. Check his oxygen.

Check *something*, because I did not sit in that waiting room next to Superglue Guy for forty-five minutes just to be handed a nasal spray and a pat on the head."

Dr. Stone stared at me.

Steve stared at me.

Chase farted.

Finally, the doctor let out a slow breath and nodded. "Alright. Let's check his vitals."

And just like that, I had won the *Battle of Emergency Room 4B.*

It turned out Chase was, in fact, not too unwell. A sore throat but no fever, no pneumonia, no low oxygen. It would be good to take bloods thought. A young registrar was given the task, one who looked about twelve and slightly sweaty.

He hovered nervously over Chase's tiny arm, needle in hand. "Alright, little guy, let's find that vein..." he mumbled, squinting like he was trying to solve a Rubik's cube. One attempt. Nope. Two attempts. Chase screamed. Three. My blood pressure skyrocketed. By the fifth failed jab, I was seriously considering snatching the needle and doing it myself when a senior doctor swooped in like a medical Gandalf.

"Enough," he said, taking Chase with the confidence of a man who had seen some things. "We'll go for a scalp vein." *A what now?* Before I could protest, he expertly slid the needle into Chase's head like it was no big deal. Chase, surprisingly, calmed down. I, on the other hand, nearly passed out. "Perfect," the doctor said, securing the line. Meanwhile, I reevaluated every life choice that had led me to witnessing *that.*

The doctor listened again to Chase's lungs and admitted his lungs sounded great. But that wasn't the point. The point was that I had *made them listen* and they had heard.

As we walked back out into the hospital parking lot, Steve put an arm around me. "You really went full mum mode back there."

"I *am* a mum."

"Yeah, but like... a *scary* mum."

I grinned. "Thanks."

Chase cooed, blissfully unaware of my warrior status, and we drove home—me, victorious; Steve, mildly traumatised; and Chase, completely indifferent to the fact that his mother had just declared herself Queen of the ER.

Google Doctor, Baby Edition – Diagnosing Chase (Sort of)

It was 2001. The internet was a wild, untamed place where the only thing more reliable than dial-up speed was the uncertainty of every search result. As a new mum, I was feeling pretty confident about a few things, least of which was raising a baby! I could run a business, make incredible sales, even garden and do some of those homely tasks everyone assumes comes naturally.

Sure, Chase had been a little fussy, and sure, he had this persistent cough, but I was *certain*—absolutely convinced—that I knew exactly that the 'maybe he might have CF' was definite. He had Cystic Fibrosis of that I was sure. How did I know? Well, because I Googled it, obviously.

Now, let me set the scene: I was a *new mum*—no prior baby experience, no clue what I was doing, but a *whole lot of Google*. As soon as I typed "baby with cough" into the search bar, it was as if the entire internet threw its arms around me in a giant, confusing, and often contradictory hug.

On one hand, there were sites that said, "A persistent cough could be a sign of something serious, like Cystic Fibrosis. Have you noticed a salty taste to his skin? Does he have difficulty breathing? Is he also building a small, but very adorable, personal empire of nappies?" I nodded solemnly. Yes, yes, and yes. Chase definitely could build an empire of nappies if we had the time.

But then, of course, there were other sites—oh, the other sites—that went in the *exact* opposite direction. "Is your baby having trouble breathing? Could be allergies. Or just a cold. Probably just a cold. Everyone gets colds. Babies get colds. It's no big deal. Cystic Fibrosis? *Ha*! Please. He's probably just teething. Or maybe he's allergic to his own baby socks. Who can say?"

Confused but empowered, I knew I had to dive deeper.

I opened another window, where an overly enthusiastic web forum had mothers sharing their "just in case" lists. "Trust your instincts!" they all screamed, like some kind of online cult. "It's better to be safe than sorry!" So here I was, clicking through forums with titles like, "My Baby Has Cystic Fibrosis and I Am Totally Fine Now," and "Don't Worry! It's Just a Runny Nose." Of course, one mother's version of "totally fine" included a daily regimen of medications that could make an old person cry and breathing treatments that sounded like they were straight out of a sci-fi movie. The other mother was like, "Yep, totally normal, just a *very persistent* cold." I didn't know which way was up. All I knew was that if my baby had CF, it was probably *definitely* worse than a cold.

But wait, the internet wasn't done with me yet.

There was the one site that told me, with complete certainty, that babies with Cystic Fibrosis should not be allowed to play with rubber ducks in the bath. "Rubber ducks can harbour bacteria, which is dangerous for CF kids," it warned. Now, mind you, I had yet to give my six-week-old a rubber duck, but I immediately pictured him staring into the abyss of a bath tub filled with toxic, bacteria-infested, life-ending plastic ducks. I Googled "What to do if your baby looks at a rubber duck," but the search results were disappointingly blank.

To add to the chaos, there was a site that claimed Cystic Fibrosis was not genetic, and could happen at any random moment like an unfortunate surprise from the universe. So, I was left wondering: did I catch it like a cold? Was I *maybe* born with it, like the worst genetic gift in history? Had I, in some alternate universe, been exposed to *a CF carrier?*

And then there were the medical sites. Ah, yes. The reputable ones that sounded professional but left me just as confused. They suggested that diagnosing CF in babies was a tricky business and that even the doctors weren't sure half the time. A page highlighted the detail of the upcoming sweat test and a genetic test—two things I had never heard of in my life until a couple of weeks ago. A sweat test? Was that a thing? I had pictured someone sticking my newborn under a heat lamp, and him just sweating his tiny baby body into oblivion, all for the sake of confirming if he had some mystery illness that only scientists knew about.

Finally, there was a site that highlighted the outcomes of CF, sober reading I can tell you. Maybe he would make five, thirteen if we were vigilant and lucky. Adulthood wasn't all that likely.

I closed my laptop, overwhelmed, devastated and sad and looked down at Chase. He was happily drooling on my finger, completely unaware that I was on the brink of a mental breakdown about the future of his health. His biggest concern at that moment was whether or not he could fit my whole finger into his mouth.

And then it hit me: maybe I was just being a dramatic first-time mum. Maybe, just maybe, Chase was just a baby who *did* have a cough, but that was also totally normal. After all, who could trust the internet when one site said I should be concerned about rubber ducks and another told me my baby would be perfectly fine?

I looked at him again, sighed, and reminded myself that babies were like little mystery boxes with a *lot* of confusing instructions. Maybe I didn't know what I was doing yet, but at least I had learned one thing that day: next time I Google symptoms, I'm going straight to WebMD and pretending I never saw the rubber duck warning.

The Sweat Test: The Most Glamorous "Science Experiment" I Never Wanted to Be a Part Of

The day we were finally going to the CF Outpatient ward for the first time, I was a ball of nerves. I'd imagined it for weeks. The hospital. The doctors. The nurses. The fluorescent lights. The clean, clinical smell of... hospital. It felt like I was about to enter some sort of medical dungeon where they'd make me sign away my sanity in exchange for a few mysterious tests.

I had built it up in my mind to be something straight out of a medical thriller. You know, the kind where the protagonist walks down long, sterile hallways with ominous music playing in the background, uncertain whether they're going to be subjected to some untested, high-tech procedure that would *definitely* involve a lot of flashing lights, beeping machines, and maybe a lab assistant wearing oversized glasses. I was *ready*. Or at least, I thought I was.

We arrived, and after passing through a maze of sterile hallways (they always look the same, don't they?), we found the CF outpatient ward. The door opened, and I half-expected to be greeted by a team of doctors in white lab coats, all standing in a perfect line with clipboards. Instead, there was a very normal receptionist and a few regular-looking nurses chatting like they had just walked out of a lunch break. No dramatic music. No high-tech beeping. No *intriguing medical assistants* giving me concerned glances.

"Well, okay," I thought to myself, "maybe the drama comes later."

We were ushered into a small, modest exam room, and I sat down with Chase, trying to maintain some semblance of composure. After a few minutes, a nurse came in and asked me to sign a few forms. All very standard, very... non-terrifying. Then she said those words I had heard over and over in my mental soundtrack: "We're going to do the sweat test today."

I braced myself.

Now, that picture I had built up in my mind of the "sweat test" being some high-stakes medical procedure where they hook m baby up to an intricate system of tubes, electrodes, and mysterious substances. In my mind, it was like they were going to put Chase through some kind of sweat-inducing gauntlet of doom. I imagined little beads of sweat being collected on microscopic glass slides that were then sent off to a remote laboratory, where scientists in white lab coats would examine them under high-powered microscopes, murmuring to each other in a foreign language as they debated the results.

I mean, sweat. It had to be complicated, right?

The nurse, clearly unaware of the movie I'd been starring in for the last few weeks, simply smiled at me and said, "Okay, let me explain how this works. We're going to apply a small patch to his arm that makes him sweat. Then we'll collect the sweat in a little tube. It'll take about 30 minutes."

My mind froze for a second. "Wait... that's it? That's the big, dramatic sweat test?"

I had expected to be thrust into a lab, locked inside some high-tech futuristic chamber where the room temperature was cranked up to 95 degrees and I would be forced to watch as Chase melted into a puddle of baby sweat while machines hummed around us. Instead, I was being told that it was literally just a small patch, and then we would just *wait*.

A small patch. A little sweat. No lasers. No flashing lights. No dramatic music.

"Is that... is that it?" I asked, half expecting her to laugh and pull out some hidden, ridiculously complicated equipment from behind her back.

She nodded, as if it was the most normal thing in the world. "Yep. Pretty straightforward."

My brain was still trying to process the understatement of the century.

So, there I was, watching as the nurse calmly placed a tiny, almost adorable-looking patch on Chase's arm. She attached it with a little piece of tape, and then we were told to wait. That was it. No grand, complicated spectacle. No moving parts. No suspenseful slow-mo close-ups of the patch being applied. Just a quiet, simple test that involved letting Chase sweat for half an hour.

Half an hour. That was my big, dramatic procedure.

We spent the next few minutes just hanging out, Chase gurgling and cooing at me, his little arm decorated with what appeared to be a patch made from nothing more than medical-grade tape and some kind of tiny absorbent material. I even tried to take a picture of it, but my phone—remember, this was 2001—had terrible resolution and I couldn't figure out how to get the flash to work. I ended up taking a blurry picture that looked like an abstract painting of a baby's arm.

It was a bizarrely calm experience. There was no beeping, no panic, no overcomplicated medical jargon. The worst part of the whole thing was waiting for the sweat to accumulate, which gave me plenty of time to mentally unpack my previously overcomplicated vision of a sweat test. I mean, how did I get *so* carried away by the idea of collecting a little baby sweat?

When the test was finally over, I couldn't help but laugh at myself. I had spent the last few weeks convinced that this test was going to be the turning point in our entire medical journey—when in reality, it was just like when you renew your license. Not that exciting, not that complicated, but still, important.

Of course the story doesn't end there. We didn't leave immediately...

The Waiting Game: Refusing to Leave the Hospital

The sweat test was over. The little patch had been removed from Chase's arm, and the nurse had smiled reassuringly, telling us that the results would take some time. I tried to breathe. I tried to tell myself that everything was fine, that there was no need to panic. But as we sat there in the sterile room, with Chase cooing quietly in my arms, it hit me.

Weeks of worry. Weeks of fear and uncertainty. Weeks of sleepless nights, Googling symptoms and reading stories of parents who had walked this same path. And now, the test was done. But there was no answer.

I could feel the panic creeping in, tightening its grip on my chest. "Someone will be in touch," the nurse had said. "It might take a few days, but we'll let you know as soon as we have the results."

A few *days*? How could I go home and wait for *days*? How could I be expected to leave the hospital without knowing what was happening to my baby? I had come this far, after all, this far down the rabbit hole of fear and research. I had read everything, I had learned so much—*too much*. I knew the signs. I knew the symptoms. I knew, deep down, what the answer was. But they weren't telling me.

Steve, was already gathering our things, ready to leave the sterile little room. He had his jacket on, and I could see the tension in his shoulders. He was done. He was ready to go home, to return to some semblance of normalcy. But I couldn't.

"No. I'm not leaving," I said firmly, standing up. "Not until I know."

Steve froze, his hand midair, about to pull the door open. He turned to me, confused. "What do you mean? The nurse said they'll contact us. It's fine. We've done everything. Let's just go home."

But I couldn't. I *knew* they knew. I had done my research. I had connected the dots. I could see the fear in their eyes, the way the nurses wouldn't meet my gaze directly, the way they avoided giving me too much information. They knew. I was sure of it. And they were waiting to give me the result when it was *official*. But the more they danced around it, the more I couldn't shake the feeling that they were trying to protect me from the worst news.

"I *cannot* go home," I said, my voice trembling despite myself. "Not until I know. I've waited long enough. I've done everything you asked. I'm not leaving without an answer."

Steve sighed, running a hand through his hair. He knew me too well—he knew I could be stubborn, but he also knew this was more than stubbornness. It was desperation. It was *fear*. His shoulders slumped. "Okay, let's just talk to someone. Just... calm down."

But there was no one. The hospital was strangely quiet, and when we asked for a doctor, we were met with the same answer: "Sorry, the doctor's not available at the moment. They'll be back later." My stomach twisted. Later? Later could be hours. Later could be *never*.

"They *can't* tell us yet," the nurse explained, almost apologetically. "They legally can't give you the results without confirming them through the proper channels. I'm really sorry."

I didn't care. I didn't care about legalities. I didn't care about processes. All I cared about was knowing whether my son had CF. Whether my son's future was going to be a hard, uphill battle or whether we had been caught in a whirlwind of parental overreaction.

I wanted an answer. I needed an answer.

So, I did what any exhausted, terrified mother might do in that moment: I refused to leave. I planted myself in the chair by the door, clutching Chase tightly to my chest, my gaze locked on the hallway outside.

Steve looked at me like I had lost my mind, and I could see the battle raging in his own head. He was calm, rational. He wanted to go home. But I was a storm, a hurricane of emotions, and there was no way I was leaving without knowing. I wasn't ready for whatever the future held, but I couldn't keep living with the unknown.

Time seemed to stretch on forever. Nurses came and went, offering little more than polite smiles and apologies. I stared at the clock on the wall, every second a weight, every minute a tiny eternity. I couldn't focus on anything except the thought of what could be happening to Chase, what could be wrong. My heart was racing, my thoughts a swirling vortex of "What ifs." What if they had already confirmed it? What if they were waiting for a specialist? What if, what if, what if?

Finally, just as I thought I might lose my grip entirely, the door opened. It wasn't a doctor. It wasn't even a nurse. It was someone from the administrative office—someone who had no answers. But as they stood there, I saw it. I saw the subtle tension in their body, the way they hesitated at the threshold.

"I... I'm sorry," they said quietly. "The doctor, the one handling your case, he's... he's not here right now. He's in another ward."

Another ward? My heart skipped a beat. The doctor I had been waiting for—the one who would have the answers—wasn't here? My mind spun. *Where was he? Why couldn't he just come in and talk to us?*

I was about to speak when they continued, their voice almost apologetic.

"The doctor... he will give you a call"

I looked at Steve, who, despite everything, seemed oddly relieved. He knew we were going to get an answer eventually. But for me, the waiting—the uncertainty—was a suffocating weight. I couldn't let go of the grip I had on this moment. I couldn't leave until I knew.

"I'm not going anywhere," I whispered, holding Chase a little tighter. "Not until I hear it from him."

The nurse was patient – more patient than I would have been. She sat beside me and said, "Donna he will call you" Something about the earnest look she gave me provided me the answer I was looking for. I nodded and stood up. We left.

What I didn't know but was to find out later was that he was with his wife. She was giving birth to their baby. A baby. His own baby. It was surreal, almost ironic. Here I was, desperate to know the fate of my son, and the very doctor I was waiting for was having the most joyous moment of his life with his own child.

He called later and with what would become his firm calm voice of reason simply said 'I cannot give you a diagnosis over the phone. I will see you next week when we will begin treatment'.

I couldn't decide whether to laugh or cry. In that moment, I understood. He was a human being, just like me, trying to balance his work with his own personal life. His wife, in labour, had to come first. I knew that. But he had called, and I knew. In that moment, nothing else mattered. Everything else had led to this. The waiting, the uncertainty, the refusal to leave—it had all led to this moment.

The time to fight for life had begun.

Welcome to the CF Club – Meds, Meetings, and Misunderstandings

The first few weeks after Chase's Cystic Fibrosis diagnosis were like stepping into an entirely new world—one where I could barely remember how to breathe, let alone navigate a maze of medications, doctor's appointments, and advice from well-meaning but often confused friends and family. It was as if we had been handed a map to a foreign country where the language was a mix of medical jargon and words like "nebulizer," "saline solution," and my personal favourite, "enzymes," all of which I'd never heard in casual conversation before.

Chase, bless his little heart, had no idea that anything was different. To him, life was pretty simple: eat, sleep, poop, and coo at us in the most adorable way possible. He had no clue that he was about to become a little medication machine in the making.

I, on the other hand, was learning a whole new vocabulary. First, there were the enzymes. The *enzymes*. Every time I thought I had them figured out—how many, when to give them, whether they should be taken before or after a feed—someone would mention *another* enzyme that did something entirely different. There was also the nebulizer, which I imagined was something from a sci-fi movie. I kept expecting it to make cool, futuristic noises like in *Star Trek*. Instead, it sounded more like a deflating balloon, and I had no idea how something that sounded so comical could be so vital to my son's health.

We quickly became well acquainted with our local pharmacist, who, at first, probably wondered if we were the *most* over-caffeinated, anxious parents he'd ever met or just some sort of emergency case that wandered in off the street. He was our lifeline—our guide to this confusing maze of prescriptions. He was *the one* who knew exactly which medication we needed, how to administer it, and, most importantly, which side effects were totally normal and which ones might require a little extra attention.

I mean, who knew that the fine art of giving a six-week-old baby multiple medications every day would be so... *complicated*? There were syringes, nebulizer cups, and even a few pill-sized items that I was convinced Chase would somehow choke on (he never did, but I'd like to think I deserve some sort of "medication prepper" medal for getting it all together). And, of course, the big question loomed: *How do you get an infant to take medication without it looking like a scene from an action movie?* Spoiler alert: you don't.

I remember the first time we had to give him his antibiotics. There we were, standing in the kitchen like we were preparing to launch a rocket. I had the syringe in hand, Steve was holding Chase, and we were both staring at our tiny, innocent child as if he had just been elected to deliver a TED Talk on the benefits of not gagging on medicine. I hesitated for a second before attempting to squirt the liquid in, only for Chase to twist his tiny face into a perfect expression of betrayal, his mouth making an exaggerated "oh no" shape as if to say, *Who dares bring this vile substance near me?*

It was a battle of wills. Chase's will to never, ever, ever let us put anything in his mouth that wasn't a bottle or his own fist, and our will to make sure he didn't end up back in the hospital. Eventually, after a few squirts of liquid medicine sprayed everywhere but in his mouth, we got the hang of it. The key? Distraction. Lots of distractions. This was when I learned that the true power of a brightly coloured toy or a well-timed song can move mountains—or at least medicate a baby.

Then there were the check-ins with friends and family. *"How's he doing?"* they'd ask, eyes wide with concern, leaning in like I was about to drop some big, dramatic update about his health. The thing was, there was no dramatic update. Chase was doing fine. *Fine.* This was the part that drove everyone—including us—absolutely nuts. Everyone expected these massive, earth-shattering moments: The big signs that his CF was affecting him in some way. But mostly, there was just... nothing.

Chase was the same weirdly skinny little baby, except now, we had this new routine. He was still *doing baby things*. And we were *doing baby things*—only now, "baby things" also included setting alarms for his meds, timing his treatments like we were trying to nail down the schedule for a military operation, and keeping a running tally of how many burps counted as "successful" digestive function for the day.

On top of that, every time someone asked how he was doing, I felt the *need* to over-explain. I couldn't just say, "Oh, he's doing fine," because that wasn't enough. I had to give them a full report. "Well, his enzymes are in check, his lung function is stable, we're managing his weight with extra calories, and he's still sleeping through the night... mostly." I was practically handing out quarterly reports at family dinners, and no one knew what to do with it. My poor sister-in-law once looked at me and said, "I think that's great, but does it mean he's... healthy? Like, really healthy?" To which I just shrugged and said, "I don't know. He *looks* healthy?"

It was strange to be *living* with Cystic Fibrosis but still feeling like I had no idea what the disease really looked like. Was Chase sick? Was he healthy? Was he doing *okay*? I kept waiting for some visible sign of the illness to show up, but instead, we just got more *routine*. Meds, nebulizers, enzymes, and visits to the pharmacist to double-check that we hadn't missed something. I had become a bit obsessed with whether or not his stool was the right colour (it was, usually), and whether he had enough energy (he did, but I could never be *sure*). It was like I had adopted a tiny, adorable little human who was also a living science experiment—and I was his very dedicated researcher.

And speaking of the pharmacist—oh, the pharmacist. We went so often, he knew us by name. He became our emergency hotline. There were times when I'd call him just to ask if a medication was supposed to *smell* like that (he assured me, yes, they all smelled awful, but that was fine). Other times, I'd find myself in the store, holding a bottle of medicine and texting him pictures. "Is this the right one? Is it okay if it's two days past the expiration date? How many doses can I *safely* skip before he mutates into a tiny, whiny monster?" He always answered with patience, even when I asked the same question for the third time in a row.

And so, we adapted. Slowly but surely, we fell into our new rhythm. It wasn't glamorous. It wasn't easy. But it was our life now, and I had learned how to be okay with it. We learned the signs that told us when Chase was doing okay: when he was eating well, when he was gaining weight, when he was smiling and kicking his legs around like a little maniac. These were the things that told us he was alright, for now.

And when those days came when we worried, we would call the pharmacist or check in with the doctors or simply look at each other and remember: we were learning. We were adapting. We might not have been experts in CF yet, but we were experts in *Chase*.

And that was all that mattered.

The Cystic Fibrosis Physiotherapy Fiasco (or How I Became a Human Bongo Drum)

When we first heard the words *Cystic Fibrosis physiotherapy*, I imagined a calm, peaceful session. In my mind, I envisioned a serene atmosphere where I'd gently pat Chase's little back in a rhythmic pattern while he cooed and giggled, blissfully unaware of the "lung-clearing" magic I was performing. Picture soft music playing in the background, a peaceful scene, and a content little baby with clear, healthy lungs.

Spoiler alert: The reality was very different.

When the physiotherapist demonstrated how to perform the percussion and lung exercises for Chase, it looked so simple. She calmly placed him on the mat, gently tapping his back in a rhythmic pattern, making it seem like a dance. Chase barely made a peep, lying there like he was enjoying a gentle massage. I thought, "Oh, this is easy. I can totally do this at home." She explained the whole process, adding a few lung exercises and some gentle tapping to break up the mucus in his lungs, and I left the appointment feeling like I had mastered the art of infant CF physiotherapy. How hard could it be to tap a baby's back, right?

Boy, was I wrong.

The first time I tried doing the percussion therapy at home, I set the stage with all the enthusiasm of a new parent who's *finally* figured something out. Chase was comfortably lying on his tummy (or so I thought), and I was ready to do my thing. I gently positioned my hands on his little back like I'd seen the physiotherapist do, preparing to tap in that perfect rhythmic pattern. I even hummed a little tune to keep things calm.

Then I tapped.

Chase's reaction was *not* the peaceful bliss I had imagined.

It started slowly—a little whimper. Then, his legs kicked out in surprise, his face contorted into an expression that looked like I had just transformed into a villain in a cartoon. I persisted, determined to follow the prescribed technique: tap-tap-tap, on each side, then the middle. Tap-tap-tap. He screamed.

I stopped. I looked down at my sweet little boy, who was now letting out a full-throated wail as if I had just entered him in a competitive sport he had no interest in participating in. "What's the matter, buddy?" I asked, as though he could tell me exactly which part of the back-tapping he found offensive. "This is for your lungs!"

He wasn't buying it.

I tried again. This time, maybe I was too hard? Maybe I was too soft? I adjusted my technique, tapping gently, then firmer, then a little softer again, trying every variation. But no matter how I did it, Chase's reaction was the same: *more screaming*. It was like my baby had been possessed by a tiny, furious protestor who would not stand for any back percussion, no matter how rhythmic.

In my head, I pictured the physiotherapist, tapping away with such calm precision, Chase lying there like an angel, giving her a look of gratitude as if to say, *Thank you for clearing my lungs, good sir*. But the reality was that, after just 30 seconds of my attempts at lung therapy, I was starting to sweat like I was in a workout class, and Chase was in the middle of a meltdown that could have rivalled a toddler tantrum at a toy store.

I needed a break. I paused for a moment to catch my breath, wiping my forehead and trying to convince myself that it was going well. In reality, the only thing I was sure of was that I was failing miserably. And then, of course, there was the inevitable moment when I began questioning everything. *Am I doing this right?* I thought. *Is this even working? Should I just call the physiotherapist and admit defeat?*

But I pushed through, figuring it had to be *me* and not the technique. After all, the physiotherapist made it look so easy.

I tried once more. This time, I'd seen that lung exercises were also a part of the therapy, and surely they'd help. I gently manoeuvred Chase's body into the position I thought was best, making sure his head was slightly elevated, and began the slow process of helping him with a bit of gentle chest compression. Maybe if I mixed up the back percussion with some gentle belly rubs, he'd be calmer?

Again, the wailing returned. Louder. I swear the sound was now coming from somewhere deep in his tiny soul, as if he was trying to warn me that I had broken some cosmic baby rule. Meanwhile, I was holding him like a little football, rocking him back and forth, attempting to tap with more "compassion" than technique. But I was beginning to suspect that my *feelings* weren't exactly helping clear his lungs.

I checked the clock: five minutes in. Five *minutes*. I was already mentally preparing myself to call in the cavalry—my husband, Steve. He could help, right? We'd take turns. Maybe we needed to approach this like a tag-team sport. So, I called out to him, "Steve! It's not working!" Of course, Steve, ever the optimist, came in full of hope and excitement, and his suggestion? "Maybe you should try a different song while you do it?"

Sure. Why not add *musical performance* into the mix? I began *tapping* and *singing* in an attempt to create the calmest, most soothing baby lung therapy experience ever. I felt like a circus performer, tapping, singing, bouncing, and trying to keep my tiny son's body from twisting into pretzel-like shapes from sheer frustration. I was convinced he'd leave a permanent imprint on the mat from how much he squirmed.

But no. Chase was having none of it.

Finally, after what seemed like a *lifetime*, I laid him down, exhausted and defeated, his face still scrunched in disbelief at what had just transpired. I wasn't sure if I had successfully cleared any mucus or just made him really mad.

I took a deep breath, trying to keep my composure, and gently kissed his forehead. "Well, buddy," I muttered. "We'll try again tomorrow."

The thing about CF physiotherapy is that, like everything with this whole journey, it doesn't go according to plan. It isn't always smooth. It doesn't always have the calm, serene moments I imagined. But we push through it. And even though I may not have been a back percussion prodigy that day, at least I tried. And Chase—well, he eventually forgave me. Or at least, he stopped crying.

The moral of the story? Lung-clearing exercises for a two-month-old baby are not glamorous. You won't be serenading your infant to sleep with lullabies while gently clearing their lungs. Instead, you might find yourself looking like a circus act. But that's okay, because in the end, you're doing the best you can—and so is your baby.

I just hoped that one day, when he was old enough to understand, Chase would say, "Thanks, Mum. I totally owe you for those lung exercises. You're my hero... even if you looked like a crazy lady."

It was only when he was a few months older that we learned he also had Tracheomalacia. Tracheomalacia in a newborn occurs when the cartilage in the windpipe, or trachea, has not developed properly. Instead of being rigid, the walls of the trachea are floppy, resulting in breathing difficulties soon after birth. This is why when he was laying down he couldn't breathe, he couldn't tell me either. No wonder he screamed!

This was one of the first areas of Chases care that I began to question quite early on. Doing something that made your baby scream even if it is meant to make them better was too much for this mum. We learned to improvise with me holding him and jumping. Possibly not a effective but it was something. Over the years physio became kangaroo jumps around the house, full on belly laughter, trampolining and sports. These days it is dance and the odd footy game. Anything to keep those rosy bellows full of life giving oxygen!

The Toddler Years - Living in the Routine That Became Our Life

When Chase turned into a toddler, I began to realise that our lives had fallen into a rhythm that was completely different from what I'd imagined for him—and certainly not what I'd imagined for *me*. At first, we had all these grand visions of typical toddler milestones: Chase learning to walk, maybe saying a few words, playing in the park, attending birthday parties, and having the kind of carefree toddler days you see on TV. Instead, we found ourselves navigating a world where hospital appointments at the CF Clinic became a routine that started off at every six weeks, then moved to three months, but never extended beyond that. Every time we got our hopes up that we were getting a break, Chase would catch another cold, or something would set off his lungs.

It was a world I never quite understood until I lived in it. And the strange part? It *felt* like home. We got to know the ward staff like family. We saw the same nurses, doctors, and specialists over and over again. At first, it was a bit awkward—like any new relationship—but before long, we were part of the team. They knew Chase by name, and I didn't have to explain his whole history with every visit. They could read his chart, and more than that, they could read *him*. They became our second family, and in some ways, I relied on them more than I relied on family and friends.

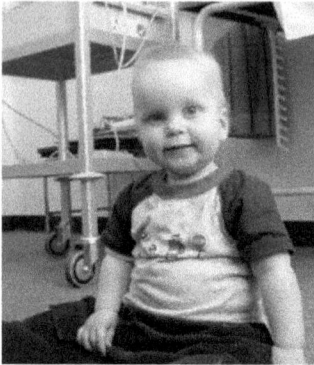

We didn't always talk about the hard stuff. We didn't need to. There were quiet nods, understanding glances, and an unspoken connection that developed over the months. Sometimes they'd ask me how I was, but most of the time, I'd brush it off and ask about Chase instead. I was learning that this wasn't just about *me* anymore; it was about *us*, and particularly about Chase.

The reality of CF and toddlerhood meant that we had to live in a way no one could have ever prepared me for. Our freezer was always stocked with homemade meals because we knew that at any moment, we'd need to prepare for a hospital stay. The constant stays—two weeks, sometimes longer—became a part of our rhythm. It was almost like running a small hospital in our own home: pumping in calories, managing medication schedules, ensuring every meal was loaded with fat and protein to help Chase thrive in spite of his illness. I'd get the calls from the clinic, and the first thing I'd do was start making arrangements. I'd take stock of the freezer, clear my work schedule, and get ready to hunker down.

And then, there were the moments when I had to find my voice—my *loud* voice, the one I never knew I had. At first, I let the doctors and specialists take the lead because I was new to this whole CF thing, but soon I began to realise that if I didn't speak up, my little boy's life would be shaped by decisions I wasn't fully involved in. I learned to ask questions, demand answers, and push back when I felt something wasn't right. I learned to stand my ground, and not just as a mom, but as a *mother on a mission*—to make sure Chase was seen first as Chase, a little boy with hopes and dreams and a future, and CF came second.

It became my mantra: *Chase first, CF second.*

It wasn't easy. There were times when I felt like I was swimming against the tide of the medical world. There were times when I doubted myself—*Am I being too much? Too loud?* But then I'd look at Chase, with his big eyes, his quirky smile, and his endless energy (when he had it), and I knew I was doing the right thing. He wasn't just a little boy with CF; he was a toddler with dreams of his own, and I wasn't going to let his illness define him in ways it didn't need to. And so, as the doctors and specialists learned to work with *us*, we learned to live with them. It wasn't always graceful, and it wasn't always smooth, but it worked.

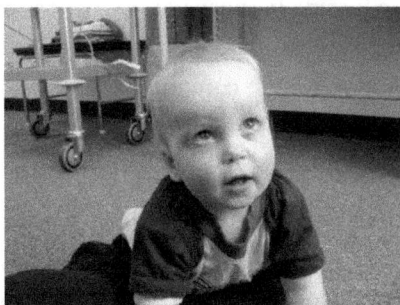

At the same time, Steve and I both had to juggle work and life. As a mum, I accepted pretty early on that working full-time while managing Chase's health was going to be a challenge. It wasn't even an option for me to go back to work full-time in the traditional sense. But I still wanted to contribute. I found ways to make a part-time schedule work and still be present for Chase. Some days felt like I was barely holding it together, but somehow, we kept going. And on the days when I did go to work, I would feel that pang of guilt, but I'd remind myself that I was doing what I could for him. I was still there, doing the best I could. And for that, I was proud.

Then, just when I thought life had settled into some kind of rhythm, we faced the most heartbreaking moment we could have imagined. Steve's dad, who adored Chase and spent every moment he could spoiling his first grandchild, passed away from cancer when Chase was only six months old. I can still feel the weight of that loss as if it were yesterday—the grief of losing someone who had been so integral to our little family, and the sadness of watching Chase grow up without his beloved Grandpa. But even in those hard moments, Chase brought light. It was through his laughter and his little milestones—his first steps, his first word, his first proper belly laugh—that we found a way to keep going.

Grief and joy lived side by side in those years. The loss of Steve's dad was a devastating blow, but life didn't stop. It couldn't. Chase needed us. And in many ways, the community we found through the CF Clinic became our second family, helping to prop us up when we needed it the most.

Around this time, I found myself getting more involved with the local CF association. It wasn't enough to just sit back and wait for answers from doctors or wait for research to find its way into our lives. I was determined to help raise awareness, to make people see what this disease could do, and to make sure that no one—no other parent—felt as isolated as I did when we first received Chase's diagnosis. I used my voice to help raise much-needed funds for research, education, and support for families going through the same thing. I couldn't fix CF. I couldn't cure Chase. But I could make sure the world was more aware of this deadly, awful disease, and I could help others who were facing the same challenges.

There were the boredom buster bags for the kids on the ward. Travelling to Auckland to meet the CEO of the Warehouses EA one day, meant we travelled back with a car load of samples and end of lines all waiting for a child to explore. There was the fabulous Drive In Movie we organised in a country that simply doesn't have a drive in movie space. It involved a crane, large screen and car radios. There was popcorn and candy floss. I don't even remember the movie but it was fun and a chance for one young man with CF to enjoy life before he passed away not long after the movie.

It wasn't glamorous. It wasn't easy. And most days, I was just trying to keep up. But the world started to see that CF wasn't just a condition. It was a fight. And we were in it together.

As the years passed, Chase continued to be our little miracle. He grew, as all toddlers do, into a stubborn, funny, and incredibly determined little boy who refused to let anything stop him. He was so much more than just his condition. And every day, I was reminded that while CF would always be a part of his life, it would never define him.

I had found my voice for Chase, and in doing so, I realised I had also found my voice for myself. And in that voice, I found the strength to face whatever came our way.

The Silent Hallways - The Isolation of CF

There's a strange kind of silence that hangs over the hospital ward. It's not the silence of peace, or calm, but the heavy, suffocating silence of knowing what's happening behind the walls. A hum of medical machinery, the shuffle of nurses' feet, the soft murmur of other parents speaking in low voices, as if the weight of the world were pressing in on us, forcing our conversations to be hushed, careful.

As I walked the sterile hallways, a part of me couldn't help but feel the presence of the other families—families like ours, navigating the very same storm, with children facing the same challenges. But that was all it was—the *feeling* of others. The reality was that, according to the new hospital rules, we couldn't connect. We couldn't talk. We couldn't even make eye contact in the waiting rooms without being mindful of the invisible line that separated us.

It was a rule that came from a good place, designed to minimise the risk of cross-infection. As if the weight of the disease wasn't enough, now we had the added burden of knowing that every person with CF was a potential risk to someone else's child. Families who once bonded over shared experiences at CF camps, those weekend getaways where we could finally speak openly with others who understood, now had to live in isolation. It felt like the very community that had supported us for so long had been pulled away, leaving us all to float in the same sea, but each in our own little boat.

I would see the other children on the ward—some of them looked just like Chase, small, tired, and strong all at once—and I couldn't help but wonder if they were thinking the same things I was. Chase, in his toddler innocence, didn't understand it, but I could see the subtle glances exchanged across rooms. Kids would look at each other, maybe in passing or when they crossed paths in the hallway, and for just a moment, I thought they recognised something in one another. Something familiar. A silent understanding. The weight they carried. The fact that, even though they were *living*, they were living in a way that not many other children could relate to.

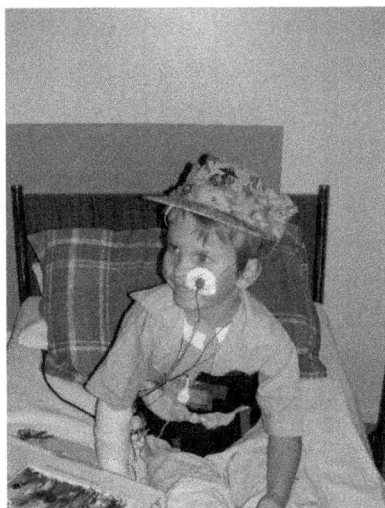

We lived in a strange kind of denial during those early years. It wasn't that we ignored what was happening—it was more that we focused so much on the day-to-day routine of medications, hospital stays, and appointments that we didn't have the energy to think beyond it. The goal was always to get through it. To get well enough to go home. We didn't have time for existential questions.

But as a mum, I couldn't ignore the feeling of isolation that crept in. I was a part of a community that I couldn't touch, couldn't really connect with. It was as if we were all part of a club no one had asked to join. And still, in the midst of that silence, we had moments—moments with other parents in the hospital rooms, those quiet conversations in the corridors where we would talk about our kids, our lives, our challenges.

I remember meeting one mother, a woman whose face had been marked with years of experience. She had two children with CF, and as we spoke about our lives, she shared the quiet pain of living with a diagnosis that was ever-present, never fading. I learned that her mother had baked our wedding cake just two years before, an unassuming but beautiful cake that marked the happiest day of my life. Yet here we were, strangers, sharing stories of how our children fought every day for breath, for life, for a future.

Her two children had both passed away too young. A part of me felt a chill when I heard those words, the harsh reality of what CF could do. The loss was too much. It was a weight that hung in the air between us, a reminder of the fragility of life. The world could feel so small when we shared those stories, so incredibly small, and yet so unbearably vast in its sorrow.

The heartbreak of losing a child is a wound that never quite heals, but it's also something that connects us, as parents of children with CF, in ways that no one else can fully understand. I felt, in that moment, the power of community. Not the kind that comes with happy faces or group gatherings, but the kind that exists in the shared grief and silent strength of knowing what it means to have a child who may not get to grow up in the way we all hoped.

CF, in many ways, can be inspiring. The resilience of the children, their ability to keep going despite the constant battles their bodies are fighting, is nothing short of incredible. But the reality of it—of the endless hospital visits, the treatments, the unrelenting pressure to be hopeful, even when all you want is for things to be "normal"—can be heartbreaking. It is a double-edged sword: the inspiration is born from the pain, and that pain never truly leaves you.

We were learning how to live within the confines of this disease, how to make our peace with it. But sometimes, it felt like our lives had been divided in two—there was life *before* CF, and there was life *after*. And after that diagnosis, it felt like everything was different. The world shifted, and we had to adapt, but in adapting, we also found our strength.

Even as we continued to live through the hospital stays, the nebulizers, the routines of breathing treatments, and the endless rounds of antibiotics, we also discovered the quiet moments of grace. The moments when Chase would smile after a rough treatment, or laugh in the face of yet another hospital visit. The way his resilience showed, even as he didn't fully understand the weight of what he was carrying.

In the silence of the ward, surrounded by the isolation that CF imposed on us, there were still those moments of connection—the quiet moments between parents, the understanding without words. And in those moments, there was strength. There was an unspoken solidarity between us, a knowledge that, though we couldn't always be with others who shared our experience, we weren't really alone.

And as I looked at my son, this tiny boy who carried so much, I found the courage to keep going. Even when the world seemed heavy, and the isolation felt endless, there was hope. There was always hope. And in that hope, we found our way forward, one step at a time.

The Decision That Would Change Everything

As parents, we all like to think that we're doing everything we can to protect our children. We do the research, we ask the tough questions, and we try to make the right choices—decisions that will keep them healthy, happy, and thriving. But sometimes, the decision we think is best turns out to be the hardest one to live with.

It was when Chase was still just a baby, around four months old, that we faced one of those decisions. It came down to something that seemed so reasonable at the time, but looking back, I wonder if I should have paused, questioned it more, and trusted my gut a little harder. But there we were, in the whirlwind of hospital appointments, constant treatments, and the never-ending cycle of "what's next," and we were offered a chance—a *chance* to help advance medical knowledge.

There was a medical trial we were asked to consider. The trial had two arms: the first was the standard process of guessing, the one we'd been living with up until now—treating symptoms, watching Chase's body respond, hoping for the best. The second arm was a little more invasive: it involved a bronchoscopy. Now, for those of you who are not intimately familiar with the world of CF, a bronchoscopy is a procedure where a small camera is threaded into the airways to identify any specific bacterial infections, and also to remove excess mucus and fluid. Essentially, it's a way to look inside the lungs when symptoms persist despite treatment, and a way to clean out the gunk that CF so often deposits in the lungs. If a sputum sample couldn't be collected, or if the symptoms—like Chase's incessant moist cough and shortness of breath—weren't responding to medication, this procedure was the next step.

At the time, I wasn't fully aware of the gravity of what that choice meant. It seemed like a step forward. A way to get ahead of the curve, to know exactly what was going on inside Chase's lungs. If we could find out what was causing the problems early enough, maybe we could fix it before it turned into something worse. Maybe we could make sure Chase didn't get too sick. Maybe we could have some control in this chaotic world of uncertainty.

But the truth is, bronchoscopy is a procedure that requires anaesthesia. It's not a small thing. They have to sedate the baby, perform the procedure, and then let them wake up in recovery. Each time Chase got sick, this would become part of the routine. Every single time he needed a procedure done, they'd wheel him away, and I'd have to sit there—clutching my hands, trying not to fall apart—while they worked to clear out his lungs.

And so, we agreed. We agreed to give Chase a chance to be part of this trial, to be in the bronchoscopy arm. We didn't know it at the time, but that decision would set the tone for so many of the hardest moments in the next few years.

Chase's first bronchoscopy was in January 2022, when he was just four months old. I remember it so clearly—the cold hospital room, the strange feeling of helplessness as we signed the papers, knowing that we were about to put our little boy through something that, while necessary, was far from easy. I tried to steel myself for what was coming. I tried to convince myself that it was the right choice, that we were doing the best thing for Chase, that this was how we'd fight CF—by staying ahead of it.

But the reality hit like a ton of bricks the first time we had to hand Chase over for the procedure. The nurses took him from my arms, and I stood there, frozen for a moment, watching them wheel him away. It wasn't the anaesthesia that terrified me. It was the idea that every time he got sick—every cough, every wheeze, every fever—this would be our new reality. It was the fact that my baby would be subjected to this invasive procedure over and over again, and that we had agreed to it without fully understanding how much it would wear on him. On *me.*

The hospital stays were short, and every time Chase was admitted, we knew what to expect. The routine of the bronchoscopy became a familiar, albeit dreaded, part of our lives. As much as we tried to manage the idea that it was just another step in keeping Chase healthy, it wore on us. The recovery periods, the uncertainty of each procedure, the constant question of *Is this enough?* It was exhausting, emotionally and physically. And each time I would go into the theatre with him helping calm him as they put the mask over his face, part of me wondered if I had made the right decision.

In the beginning, I told myself I could handle it. I convinced myself that I was doing this for Chase, that this was what needed to happen. But as the months went by, as Chase got older and started to develop his own personality, I started to feel the weight of it all more. I saw how much it affected him. He would cry when the doctors came into the room, even though they tried to be gentle. He would look up at me with those big, trusting eyes as if asking, *Why are you letting them do this to me?*

And it wasn't just the physical toll on him; it was the emotional toll it took on *us.* The weight of knowing that every time Chase caught a cold or started to show signs of a flare-up, we would have to repeat the process. It felt like there was no end in sight, no finish line where we could finally say, "Okay, we're done."

Looking back now, as I sit here and reflect on those first years, I realise that, as much as I wanted to believe I was making the best choice, I was also caught in a system where the options were limited. In my effort to give Chase the best chance at a normal life, I had unknowingly set us on a path that would become more challenging than I had ever imagined.

I strongly believe that regardless of what the Doctors said at the time, babies should never have an anaesthetic unless they are in mortal danger. This for me at least was reinforced as truth when 12 years later a further study was done that we also participated in – whether anaesthetics in young children with CF had any impact on their psychological or intellectual outcomes. That study's results which started in 2014 have yet to be released.

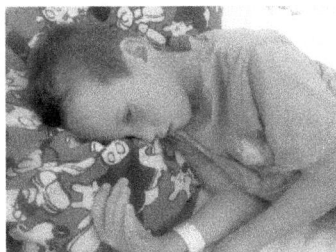

I didn't know then, but I know now, that sometimes, even with the best of intentions, the decisions we make as parents are not always the right ones. The road ahead is unpredictable, and some of the choices we make are ones we come to regret.

But one thing I've learned is that, as parents, we do the best we can with the information we have at the time. We make decisions out of love, out of fear, out of hope. And sometimes, even when things don't go as planned, those decisions are the ones that teach us the most about ourselves, about our children, and about the incredible strength we carry within us.

So, I stand here now, looking at Chase, watching him live his best life and face challenges I never could have imagined, and I know that even though I regret some of the choices we made along the way, I would do it all over again for him. Because in the end, this journey is his, and I'll continue to fight beside him, no matter what path we take.

The Great Chase – Discovering the World, One Snack at a Time

Chase was ready to take on the world. Well, a very small, carefully monitored, hand-sanitized portion of the world—but still, it was progress!

At home, we had settled into our routine of medications, physio, and enough calorie counting to qualify me for a job as a high-performance sports dietitian (if only stuffing my child with butter and coconut oil counted as a professional skill). But Chase needed more. He needed people, adventure, and a break from my overly enthusiastic meal-planning. Enter Tracy.

Tracy was a home-based caregiver, but more importantly, she was a *miracle worker.* From the moment Chase waddled into her care, he became part of her family. He was the much-loved extra child, the tiny tornado of energy who charmed his way into everyone's hearts. While I was at work, Tracy took on the never-ending mission of keeping Chase entertained, fed, and, most importantly, *gaining weight.* I'd drop him off in the morning with a bag full of enzyme capsules, an inhaler, and an enthusiastic reminder to "encourage calories!" and by pick-up time, she'd be handing me back a sticky, giggling toddler with more food on his face than in his stomach—but full of love, laughter, and just enough weight gain to keep the dietitians from panicking.

Despite our best efforts, hospital stays were still part of the routine. But they seemed to have a schedule of their own—specifically, around Easter and his birthday in September. Every year, without fail, just as we were gearing up for chocolate-fuelled chaos or a cake-filled birthday celebration, Chase would start showing signs of another respiratory infection. I blamed the change of seasons, the ever-present sniffles that other kids would shake off but, for Chase, turned into a ticket straight to the hospital. It was like his lungs had an *alarm system* for special occasions.

But there is always a silver lining – Easter generally meant we got to watch the Hot Air Balloon display from the window, safely and with one of the best views. September meant spending Chases birthday hanging out on the ward with just a few extra fun activities with the staff.

By now, we had adjusted to the hospital routine. We knew the nurses by name, and the ward staff knew Chase's favourite cartoons. I had a freezer permanently stocked with homemade meals, ready to grab when we got the inevitable call saying, *"Better come in, we need to admit him."* I was no longer just a mum—I was a *hospital warrior*, armed with snacks, spare clothes, and enough antibacterial wipes to sterilise an entire operating room.

The Great Tube Disaster of Christmas

One of the biggest changes came when Chase had to get a 'Mickey' button—a gastrostomy tube to help supplement his calorie intake. It was a big step, but given how much of my day was spent obsessing over his weight, I was actually relieved. Now, no matter what, Chase would get the nutrients he needed. Easy, right? HA!

The procedure went smoothly, but because this was *our* life, things couldn't stay that way. Just before Christmas—when, of course, every supplier of medical equipment had gone on their well-deserved holiday break—the button *fell out.* This left us with a *giant* hole in Chase's stomach, a gaping little portal to his insides that needed urgent fixing.

Enter the *Doctor Who Clearly Had No Idea What He Was Doing.* This well-meaning but utterly clueless man took one look at the situation and, in his infinite wisdom, inserted a *drainage tube.* Not a replacement feeding button, not something properly designed to hold things in place. A *drainage* tube. His brilliant plan? *"Just clamp it shut until we can order the proper replacement after Christmas."*

Well, dear reader, as it turns out, simply *clamping* a drainage tube is not a foolproof way to prevent stomach contents from escaping. Every single meal turned into a gross, leaky mess. Chase would eat, and within minutes, his stomach contents would gleefully pour out onto his clothes, the couch, the floor— *everywhere.* I spent two weeks running around with towels, spare outfits, and a look of sheer horror every time we attempted another meal. It was like living inside a science experiment gone horribly, disgustingly wrong. Add to this granularisation around Chases mickey button site. Granulation describes the appearance of red, bumpy tissue in the wound bed as the wound heals. This bumpy appearance is the visible tops of the new capillary loops as a new vascular supply develops to serve the newly forming tissue with oxygen and nutrient. It was often oozing, making for an uncomfortable experience. We all have a certain amount of Staphylococcus on our bodies. The last thing we need was for Chase to get it inside his body. To resolve the issue, we were prescribed Silver Sticks.

Silver nitrate kills bacteria and other microorganisms in the wound, preventing infection and promoting tissue regeneration. Reduction of Infection: Over the following days to weeks, the antimicrobial properties of silver nitrate help reduce the risk of infection and minimize bacterial colonisation in the wound. They also burn. So for a few weeks I would burn Chases skin in order to get it to heal without infection. It was an awful time!

By the time the *actual* Mickey button was finally available, I practically tackled the medical supplier with gratitude. I had never been so happy to see a small piece of medical-grade plastic in my life. At this point in time, I was simply the observer as it was replaced. In years to come I would be the regular changer. That was until we moved to Australia where it was only to be done by a medical professional as we mere mums could not be trusted to do it.

In NZ, it was an entirely different philosophy – the more we mums could do the more we could alleviate the healthcare system. It would take many years for me to successfully navigate the Australian health care system... actually I simply got kicked out when Chase became an adult.. although in recent times I have noted that it is drawing me back in...apparently for advice as I might know a thing or two about Chase.. who'd figure!

The Calorie Wars

If there was one ongoing battle in our house, it was the *War of the Calories.* Keeping Chase's weight up was a full-time job. It still is. He is sitting here right now on his 7th meal of the day!

Forget picky eating—this was a whole new level of food obsession. The dietitians would give me pep talks: "Just sneak extra calories into his food! Make everything high-fat! Get creative!" And oh, *I did.*

Coconut oil? Yep, that went into EVERYTHING. Porridge, mashed potatoes, scrambled eggs—if it could be mixed, melted, or blended, I was putting coconut oil in it. Butter? Chase ate more butter than any two-year-old should legally be allowed to consume. Cheese? If it had even a vague resemblance to food, I covered it in cheese. I was *this close* to sneaking double cream into his water bottle. There was the homemade pate which Chase simply loved on toast .. until he didn't. Pasta that made you go faster smothered in three kinds of cheese. A snack box well within his reach and weekly outings to Maccas, KFC, pizza... you get the picture..? Chase's favourite food – vegetables.

Yep, for me this vege hating mum, I was to be found in the kitchen with veges galore. Generally covered in cheese, cheese sauce, or roasted and drowning in gravy I made this kid eat! He would munch away happily and yet the weight never seemed to be enough to get him out of the 5th percentile in terms of BNI! A telltale sign of him becoming unwell, would be obvious to me as his mum. He could be found running down the hallway sans nappy and his butt perfectly round in the morning seemed to be this sagging pocket of skin by afternoon. He would cough and I would see his tiny chest sink even further in. His laughter betrayed his unwellness.

I knew gaining weight gave us a fighting chance against the demon of CF.

However, despite my best efforts, Chase, being the independent little rascal he was, had no interest in my calorie-boosting sorcery. He ate what he wanted, when he wanted, and no amount of desperate pleading, airplane noises, or *"Look, it's a magical cheese castle!"* trickery could change his mind.

Through it all, I learned to laugh. Because honestly, what else can you do when you're standing in the middle of your kitchen at 2 AM, spooning melted butter into a tiny bowl of mashed potatoe, praying that this *one extra mouthful* will make a difference?

In the end, we found our rhythm. Chase grew, on his terms, in his way. Tracy remained his second mum, giving him a home away from home filled with love and cuddles. Hospital stays became part of our *weirdly normal* life, and I mastered the art of sneaking calories into food in ways that would impress even the most seasoned chef.

Life with Chase was never predictable, never easy—but it was always *his*. And no matter what challenges CF threw our way, we were in it together. With coconut oil, far too much cheese, and a whole lot of love.

The Butterfly Takes Flight – Chase Goes to Kindergarten

Deciding to send Chase to kindergarten felt a little like throwing a delicate yet determined butterfly into a wind tunnel. On one hand, we wanted him to experience everything childhood had to offer—messy painting, sandpit adventures, the joy of sticky fingers and chaotic group play. On the other hand... *germs*. So many germs. An entire petri dish of tiny, sneezy, sniffling children just *waiting* to share their latest viral sensation.

But Chase was ready—well, as ready as he ever would be. His world had been small for so long, wrapped in the safe cocoon of home, hospital, and Tracy's care. It was time to spread his wings.

We had always known Chase was a little different. Not in a way that worried us—more in a way that made us laugh and shake our heads in wonder. He had the attention span of a gnat. He could be mid-sentence (well, mid-babble) and suddenly become *entirely* distracted by a single hair on the floor. *A single hair. From across the room.* I swear, if CSI ever needed a toddler with the forensic abilities of a crime-scene investigator, Chase was their guy.

He took his time with milestones. Sitting up unaided? Nearly a year. Walking? Oh, no rush—he waited a solid *18 months* before deciding to give that a go. We had a neurodevelopmental therapist visit us when he was nine months old, a lovely woman who spent an exhausting *four hours* assessing him, only to conclude, "Do more physio. He'll catch up."

Ah yes, *he'll catch up.*

We heard that phrase a lot. *He'll catch up* became the comforting yet vague promise that dangled before us, just out of reach. And to be fair, he did—just on his own timeline. Even today, he's still playing catch-up in some ways, but back then, we had no idea what was ahead. All we saw was a bright, beaming little boy who floated through life like a butterfly—flitting from one thing to another, smiling as he went.

Walking into that kindergarten for the first time was like stepping into another universe—one filled with chaos, laughter, and a constant hum of activity. It was overwhelming, exciting, and *terrifying*. For me, not him. Chase? He strolled in like he owned the place. He wouldn't need the reassurance of a blankie like his younger brother. He wouldn't cry when I left. In fact, he never cried when I left the room, the hospital the shop – anywhere! He was so involved in the moment I was secondary to his thoughts. It was a warning sign over our bow that we did not read nor understand.

The teachers fell for him immediately. How could they not? He was the child who *lived in the moment*, soaking up every sound, every colour, every bit of joy that came his way. He wasn't the kid sitting neatly in a circle or following instructions with precision (*let's be real—that was never going to happen*), but he was the one who would stop everything just to enjoy the feel of paint between his fingers or the way the light made a rainbow through the classroom window. He made friends. He would dress up. He was enthralled at the activities, the energy and the action.

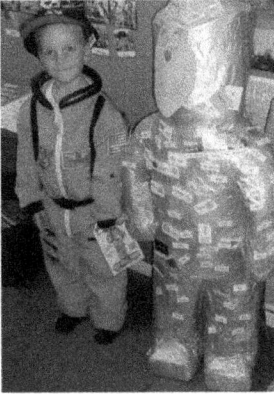

His gross and fine motor skills weren't quite on par with the other kids, but that didn't stop him from joining in. He just did things *his way*. Running? More of an enthusiastic shuffle. Cutting with scissors? More like *aggressively mauling paper until it resembled modern art*. But no one cared, because Chase brought something else to that classroom—pure, unfiltered joy.

We had sent Chase to kindergarten hoping it would help him grow, but what we hadn't expected was how much he would impact *others*.

His teachers saw it first. That sparkle, that *something special* about him. He wasn't just a child with extra challenges; he was a child who made people *feel*. He reminded them to slow down, to appreciate the small things, to laugh at the ridiculous and find joy in the simple.

And his classmates? Some adored him. Some didn't. Sure, he might have been a little slower, a little different, but he was *Chase*. The one who would giggle at the sound of Velcro, who would stop mid-play to stare in wonder at a butterfly landing nearby. The one

69

who didn't care about keeping up—because he was too busy just *being*. There was a young man that didn't get him, not at the start. He was too different to Chase. He was quiet and thoughtful. He was slight like Chase though and perhaps that's what connected them – they were mirror images of each other. The little boy was Jed. And they became best friends from kindergarten, through primary school even remaining friends after we moved to Australia. They are still mates, each with their own lives in different countries, but in touch and supporting each other as they have for 20years.

At the time, before school, even while Chase was in kindy, we didn't know about the developmental challenges that lay ahead. We didn't know about his low IQ, or the struggles with cognitive processing, or that *catching up* wasn't something that would magically happen overnight.

All we knew was that Chase was *happy*. That he was out in the world, making friends, making *ripples* in people's lives in a way only he could.

Kindergarten wasn't just the start of his education. It was the start of *his impact on the world.*

And it was my chance to hone my advocacy skills outside of the medical system. To advocate for Chases learning. The kindy team were kind, caring and supportive. I still have the folders carefully constructed by staff for each child. Chases is full of him laughing, dressed up, snotty nose looking half the size of the other children but always having fun.

I learned in his time at Kindy to help others to read the signs when he was unwell. Or to help them encourage him to eat. To help provide those firm lines and structure to allow him to stay on track. There would be the conversations of support whereby I handed over the decision making to them while Chase was there. A few tips on how to know if his mickey button might be loose and to call me. There were conversations about an impending procedure such as a port flush which Chase particularly *hated* (yes a strong word – he did hate them) and how they could distract him so he didn't overly worry.

We worked together to ensure he remained included even if he was away for a few weeks in hospital. This was an amazing team of dedicated professionals. When the kindy was threatened with closure, I was on the picket line! It did close for a year before reopening bigger and taking on more children. Chase would be at school by then, but it would provide Joshua, Chase's younger brother with the same love, care and support a number of years later.

We revisited kindy a few years back with Chase grown up alongside his younger brother. The building remained the same, and some of the staff were still there. There were new staff too. When we popped in the hugs were immediate and even the new staff commented about this young man Chase who they had heard so much about! How the staff had discovered a lot about connecting the medical world with early education. How they played a key role in helping someone like Chase gain confidence in the world outside of his home. I was to be surprised and perplexed a few months after Chase started school at home different early education and school life were!

And honestly? That was worth every single germ he picked up at Kindy.

School Days, Pies, and the Art of Controlled Chaos

Sending Chase to school wasn't just a milestone—it was a *logistical operation of epic proportions*. Forget the usual worries about packed lunches and lost jumpers; we had *medical manuals* to deliver, emergency plans to create, and a child to launch into an education system that had precisely *zero funding* to support him.

It would be like a Crash Course in Chase Management!

Our first meeting with the school staff resembled a hostage negotiation—except I was the one handing over the demands.

"Okay, so here's the deal. Chase has Cystic Fibrosis, which means he needs to take his enzymes before eating, he needs extra salt, extra calories, and basically all the food society has labelled as *bad*—so yes, if he's eating a donut and you take it away, we will have words. *Firm words.*"

Blank stares.

I continued, *"Also, if he starts coughing and can't stop, call me. If he looks unusually tired, call me. If he's wheezing, struggling to breathe, or turning a delightful shade of blue—skip calling me and dial an ambulance. And if he's about to get on the wrong bus after school, physically stop him. He will wander off, and we live in the country—so if you lose him, you're looking at a small-scale search-and-rescue mission."*

More blank stares.

"And if you're wondering why I'm explaining all this with no extra staff or support for him... well, so am I."

One of the great ironies of Chase's school experience was lunchtime. While other parents were sneaking carrot sticks into

72

their kids' meals, I was practically stuffing his backpack with high-calorie contraband. *More butter, more cheese, more everything.* But school rules dictated that *all* children had to sit down and eat their lunches *before* playing.

This was a *travesty* in Chase's world.

He didn't want to sit still and eat; he wanted to *move*. Run, jump, explore—anything but sit on a bench like a caged animal.

One day, I got a call.

"Uh, Ms. Slater Chase keeps trying to escape lunch."

"Yes. And?"

"Well, he's really *insistent* on not eating."

"That's because he thinks it's a waste of time."

Long pause. "But... he *has* to sit and eat."

I sighed. "Look, if you need him to sit, try feeding him like a tiny king. Bring him a sandwich *while* he runs. Offer him food like it's a drive-thru window. He'll eat—just not the way you want him to."

They were not amused. Chase, on the other hand, found it all hilarious.

Making friends was vital, but Chase needed some help navigating social norms—like *personal space*. His concept of boundaries was... *fluid*. If he wanted to be close to someone, he *would be close*—whether they liked it or not.

And, of course, kids can be *cruel* in that unthinking way small humans sometimes are. They quickly learned that Chase's simple outlook on life meant he was easy to manipulate.

"Chase, go poke Jack in the back."

He'd do it.

"Chase, go take Lucy's hat."

Done.

Cue teachers calling me, frustrated that Chase was "always getting into trouble."

"Do you think," I asked one particularly exasperated staff member, "that perhaps he's being *set up*?"

Silence. Then: "Oh. Well. I hadn't thought of that."

Of course they hadn't. They saw a kid who didn't always follow the rules, not the *why* behind it. Chase didn't understand that not everyone was his friend, and that terrified me. He did have Jed thought, with him and Shantel he had supporters that stood by him and up for him. Telling him to not be an idiot when he needed it and simply laughing with him when life was good.

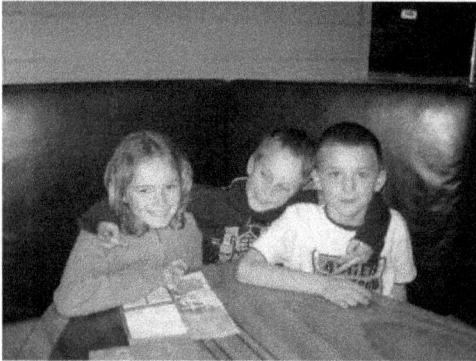

They say *never compare your child to others*.

Yeah, okay. But also? *We all do it.*

Not in a mean way—just in a *where are we on the scale of development* kind of way. And once school started, I couldn't help but notice how Chase's journey differed. Other kids were reading, writing, grasping concepts that seemed lightyears away for him. I tried to push it down, to remind myself that he was *him*—that he'd do things *his* way.

But deep down, I knew.

I knew that "he'll catch up" was wishful thinking. That this was going to be *our* version of school, not the typical one. And that scared me.

But at the same time, I knew Chase. I knew his spark, his determination, his *absolute refusal* to be anything other than *himself*. And maybe—just maybe—that was more important than any test score.

After all, the world had enough kids who could colour inside the lines.

It needed more kids like Chase.

A Different Kind of Normal

Life had settled into a rhythm. Not a *normal* rhythm, at least not by other people's standards, but our own version of normal—one that involved carefully scheduled hospital stays, a deep love-hate relationship with medical supplies, and the ever-present battle of Chase's weight.

School holidays weren't for vacations. They were for *rebuilding*.

While other families packed suitcases and road-tripped to the beach, we packed overnight bags for the hospital. Two weeks of IVs, tests, recalibrations—fixing him up just enough to send him back out into the world for another school term. It was our *pit stop*—like a race car pulling in for fresh tires and fuel before tearing off again. Only, in our case, Chase wasn't so much *tearing off* as *flitting through life like an overcaffeinated butterfly.*

Despite *everything*—the endless calorie-packed meals, the butter-laden everything, the nightly tube feeds—Chase's weight remained *the* issue. The *forever* issue.

His ever present gastrostomy tube, should have made life easier, but of course, nothing was *ever* that simple. Nightly pump feeding meant waking up *every three hours* to inject powdered enzymes down the tube so his body could actually *process* the food. That lasted until sheer exhaustion forced me to cut back to *three nights a week*—because not sleeping and then attempting to be a functioning adult at work was, shockingly, *not sustainable*.

It didn't matter how much we tried—he burned through calories like a furnace with a broken thermostat.

Through all of this, I felt a growing tension—two pulls, both demanding my attention.

The first was Chase's *life*. Not just his *health*, but his *actual life*. A *life well lived*.

We had seen too much. Too many other children—kids Chase had shared hospital corridors with—were passing away in their early teens. *Teens*. Not even *adults*. We had watched as new treatments were dangled like a carrot in front of desperate families, only to disappear before they could ever reach the children who needed them. We had to *hang on*.

And hanging on didn't just mean fighting the disease—it meant *living, experiencing, making memories*.

I wanted to make sure Chase had a life filled with adventure, with stories, with things that made him *laugh until he couldn't breathe* (though preferably not *medically*).

And so, a plan was forming in the back of my mind. A *ridiculous, possibly unachievable* plan—but one that had been inspired by a Christmas classic: *Home Alone 2: Lost in New York*.

Because what better way to live a full life than to recreate *that* adventure?

But as I started plotting this *grand* scheme, I felt the second pull growing stronger.

I wanted another child.

But not one with CF.

I loved Chase with *every fibre* of my being, but I couldn't do it again. I *couldn't*. The sleepless nights, the endless medical appointments, the terrifying uncertainty of *if*—not *when*—he would get sick again.

Steve and I talked. Debated. Questioned. How could we do this? Should we even try? Could we *ensure* another child wouldn't have CF? Was it fair to Chase, to us, to anyone?

It was a dilemma that didn't have an easy answer.

But one thing was clear.

No matter what happened, Chase's life *would* be one well lived.

The Journey to Two

Chase was nearly seven, and was our own, carefully balanced, medicalised version of normal. He was a whirlwind of energy, a butterfly of a child, flitting from one thing to the next with that ever-present smile. He had grown into a kid who saw the world through his own unique lens, always ready to make a game out of anything, but also always fighting battles most other kids never had to. He played soccer… badly. He loved kid Ironman and excelled at the running, struggled with the bike and frankly nearly drowned in the pool. But he loved it. He loved it so much and was smiling so much when he collapsed over the finish line one year at school we all yelled hooray!! Only to find a few hours later sitting in the hospital that he had full blown pneumonia and was struggling to breath! Yes he lived life!

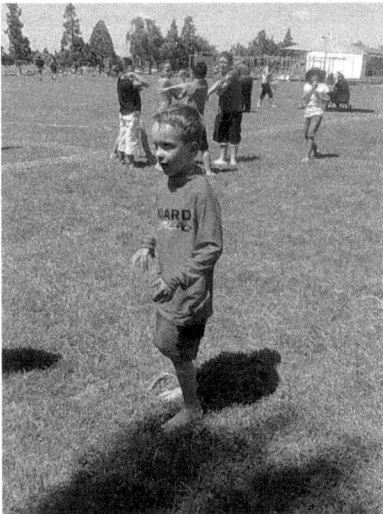

And soon, he was about to have a baby brother.

Getting to this point had been a journey. *A three-year* journey through IVF, PGD (preimplantation genetic diagnosis), and a medical system that had felt as invasive as it was rewarding.

But it would cost us.

We hadn't walked this road alone. Cameras had followed us—capturing every appointment, every decision, every tear-filled conversation. The world would see what it took, what it *really* took, to have a child *without* cystic fibrosis when both parents were carriers. The process had been relentless, stripping away any illusion of privacy.

Blood tests. Hormone injections. Scans. Needles. Failed attempts. Heartbreaking calls telling me embryos hadn't survived. The victories were small and rare, and the losses felt overwhelming. IVF wasn't just a physical battle; it was emotional warfare. And as the months turned into years, I felt myself changing.

I had always been strong—because I *had* to be. But this? This tested me in ways I hadn't expected.

I began to push Steve away.

He didn't understand the weight of it all, not the way I did. He wasn't the one being poked and prodded, the one charting every hormone level, the one enduring the crushing hope that rose and fell with every cycle. He loved me, and he loved Chase, but he couldn't *feel* it the way I did.

And then, with cameras rolling, I said the thing that would shock even myself.

I told the world that I loved Chase more than anything, but if I had another baby with cystic fibrosis—I would rather *abort* than go through it all again.

It was brutal. It was raw. It was *the truth*.

I knew what CF meant. I had lived it. I had fought alongside Chase every single day. And I couldn't do it again. Not because I didn't love him, but because I *did*.

Because I had seen the endless nights in the hospital. Because I had watched parents bury their children. Because I had spent years fighting, pushing, battling just to keep Chase here *one more day*.

How far I *would* go had been clear from the start.

But I had also discovered how far I *wouldn't* go.

The invasiveness of procedures despite the care of the medical staff became too much. Already exhausted in taking care of Chase, working and trying to be a good wife, I had nothing left to give so pulled out of the program. I was defeated.

And then I got pregnant.

As I stood on the edge of a new reality, with Chase twirling in circles in the living room, completely oblivious to the weight of the journey that had brought us here, I felt something I hadn't felt in years.

Hope.

This baby, this new life, was a symbol of everything we had fought for—not just for him, but for *us*. For Chase. For our family.

It had taken three years, relentless determination, and a medical world that had tested my very soul, but soon, Chase would have a baby brother.

And for the first time in a long time, I felt like we were about to win.

A Baby, A Bill, and a Hospital Room

Being 38 weeks pregnant is an experience in itself. Being 38 weeks pregnant *and* trapped in a hospital room with your sick child? That's a whole new level of chaos.

I was *huge*. Not just pregnant, but *planetary*. If I had to roll over in bed, it required a full strategy meeting and possibly a construction crane. And yet, here I was, waddling through the halls of the children's hospital, balancing my enormous belly while simultaneously trying to keep Chase from yanking out whatever IV they'd attached to him this time.

I should have been home, propping my swollen feet up on a pillow, enjoying those last few weeks of relative calm before a newborn turned our world upside down again. Instead, I was in my familiar spot beside Chase's hospital bed, half-heartedly attempting to sleep on one of those plastic reclining chairs designed by someone who *clearly* hated parents.

And yet, somehow, I knew it would all be okay. *Somehow.*

Of course, just before all of this, I had turned *forty*. A milestone birthday! A moment to reflect, to celebrate, to bask in the wisdom of my years!

Or, in my case, to be stuck with the bill at dinner while my husband and mother-in-law smiled sweetly across the table.

Yes, that's right. My grand *fortieth birthday celebration* consisted of a meal at my favourite restaurant, followed by the waiter *handing me* the check. I'd like to say it was a mistake, but no. Somehow, in the fine art of familial negotiations, I ended up paying for my own birthday dinner.

And the gifts? Oh, they were *spectacular*.

My mother-in-law, in a moment of true maternal wisdom, gifted me... *a set of pearls*. It was a gift I would treasure later on when I needed to feel special, or classically smart. That woman could pick a gift – sometimes it was her timing that sucked...like the time she gave me a Christmas gift to open in New York...wrapped carefully I snuck a look... thank goodness I did... it was a nail set with scissors... had I taken it on the plane – it would have been confiscated! I still have it luckily a bit worn and battered but a reminder of her.

And Steve? My *beloved* husband? The man who had shared my life, my joys, my sorrows, my love?

He bought me... nothing.

Not a card. Not a flower. Not even a passive-aggressive IOU.

But I digress.

The one gift I *did* get that year? The knowledge that baby Joshua, the little kicker currently rearranging my organs, *probably* didn't have CF. Probably.

The PGD process had been thorough, but science, for all its miracles, still left room for a tiny sliver of doubt. Until Joshua was born and we could do a gene test, there was always that whisper in the back of my mind: *What if we were wrong?*

But I had spent the last seven years worrying myself into exhaustion, and I decided—at least for now—that I would let myself believe in the "probably."

And then, suddenly, Joshua *was* here.

I had given birth via a caesarean under a general anaesthetic ,
and after a few days of meandering through postpartum
exhaustion, we were finally bringing our second son home.

It was the same, yet entirely different.

With Chase, we had walked through the door seven years
earlier with a fragile, beautiful newborn *and* a regimented medical
schedule that ruled our lives. I had become an expert in crushing
tablets in the dark, counting enzymes like a scientist on the verge of
a breakthrough, and scheduling feeds with military precision.

With Joshua?

There was... *nothing*. No medication. No alarms. No sterile
bottles filled with medical-grade calorie boosters. Just a baby. A
blissfully *normal* baby.

I had almost forgotten how to change a nappy, but—like
riding a bike—it came back to me (remembering to ensure I had
everything prior to nappy change to avoid wearing its contents!   I
had forgotten something special - the smell.

Oh, that *newborn smell*. That intoxicating, slightly milky,
slightly sweet, utterly perfect scent that made all the sleepless
nights, swollen ankles, and *fortieth birthday indignities* worth it.

For the first time in years, I could wake up in the middle of
the night and *not* have to crush medication. I could rock my baby to
sleep without worrying about whether his lungs were filling with
mucus. I could just *be* a mum, in the simplest, purest form.

And as Chase stood next to the bassinet, staring down at his
tiny, wrinkly new brother with a mix of fascination and absolute
boredom, I realised something.

Our family had changed, grown, and stretched in ways I could have never imagined. And while our life would never be "normal" in the way others defined it, this?

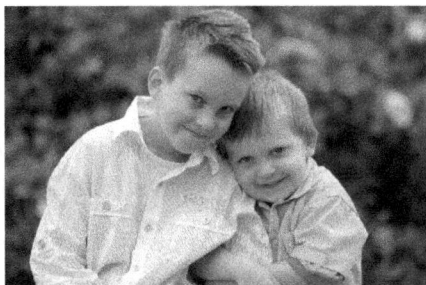

This was *our* normal. And somehow, that was enough, for now.

The Dream Begins to Form

Chase was never in a rush. Not to walk, not to talk, and certainly not to finish his homework. While other kids zoomed past him academically like Olympic sprinters, Chase preferred a leisurely stroll through the world of education, whistling as he went. If learning was a race, Chase was the guy taking scenic detours and stopping to admire the flowers. But was he worried? Absolutely not.

I, on the other hand, spent years in a constant state of panic. It wasn't just school that worried me; it was the basics of life. Like remembering to take his tablets—sometimes up to 40 a day. You'd think that by the time he had been swallowing them for over a decade, it would be second nature. You would think wrong.

"Mum, did I take my tablets?" he'd ask, standing in front of an empty blister pack.

"Well, did you?" I'd reply, staring at him intently, hoping for a sign of recognition.

"I dunno. Maybe?"

Cue my deep sigh and frantic recounting of the morning's events. You'd swear I was running a pharmaceutical inventory rather than raising a child. But Chase's ability to use what most of us take for granted—his initiative—was, let's just say, severely compromised. No number of reminders, alarms, or Post-it notes could guarantee success. If anything, the alarms just became part of the background noise of our lives, blending in with the beeping of the microwave and the occasional honk of an impatient driver outside.

I knew something wasn't right, but how do you put that into words? How do you explain that your child is bright and engaging, able to hold conversations with adults about politics or history, yet completely unable to relate to his peers? It wasn't until 2008, after Joshua's arrival, that someone else finally noticed what I had been struggling to articulate for years.

An assessment was scheduled. I sat behind the one-way glass, watching Chase navigate a series of tests designed to evaluate his cognitive abilities. What I saw was telling in that his inability to focus. The constant need to talk about the most unrelated subjects, the almost wearisome communication was our normal. What the professionals saw was clear. The diagnosis? Intellectual Disability.

I scoffed. No, that couldn't be right. Chase wasn't disabled; he was just… different. Quirky. Unconventional. A late bloomer. The kind of person who would one day surprise us all. I refused to accept it, pushing the words aside as if they were merely suggestions rather than a clinical diagnosis. It would take me another eight years to fully understand and accept it. But in the meantime, life went on.

Between managing a newborn, working to help Steve provide, and navigating the financial tightrope that is parenting, there was no time to dwell. Chase continued to exist in his own world, unbothered by grades, social norms, or the idea of "catching up."

Then one day, through one of our many casual conversations, a dream was born.

"Mum, you know Home Alone – could we go there?."

Without thinking, without planning, without realising what I had just done, I said, "Yeah, let's do this."

And just like that, the dream took hold. It wasn't just a trip anymore. It was a mission, a goal, the project of Chase's lifetime. And knowing Chase, it would be anything but straightforward.

The Art of Fundraising (or How I Became a Reluctant Hustler)

Here is the thing with agreeing to a dream.... it requires action. And dreams generally cost money. And sometimes - well at least in this case it was going to be a considerable amount of money to fly to the other side of the world .

If there was one thing I knew for sure, it was that I could not ask people for money. Not because I didn't believe in the cause—after all, it was my big mouth that had blurted out, *"Yes! Let's do this!"*—but because asking for money made me break out in hives.

Steve, being the practical one, had already decided he wasn't going on this trip, declaring, *"It should just be you and Chase to keep costs low."* Low? LOW?! We were talking about taking a child who required up to 40 tablets a day across the world to a country where even sneezing could land you with a medical bill the size of a mortgage.

The health insurance alone made my stomach drop. If Chase got sick in the US, we might as well hand over the house keys and move into a cardboard box. There was no way we could afford to cover an American hospital stay. The stakes were high, but so was my stubbornness. We were doing this, even if it meant I had to develop a whole new personality—one that could beg, barter, and borderline extort (legally, of course).

Thankfully, I wasn't alone. Friends rallied around, and we started coming up with ideas. The first? Selling kindling. It sounded simple enough. People donated wood, we packed it up, and Chase helped deliver it to customers for $10 a bundle. I should have known that "helped" was a loose term. Chase, bless him, was not built for manual labour.

Each delivery went something like this:

Me: *"Chase, grab that bundle and take it to the door."*
Chase: *"But what if a dog is there?"*
Me: *"You knock and find out."*
Chase: *"But what if the person is scary?"*
Me: *"You're not selling encyclopedias, just drop the wood and smile!"*
Chase: *"Mum, can I just supervise?"*

By "supervise," he meant sitting in the car while I did the heavy lifting.

Then his teacher, inspired by the project, decided to run a marathon to raise money. Chase, not being one for running unless it involved a buffet, took on the role of her cheerleader. He wore the title with pride, standing at the finish line holding a sign that said, *"Run Faster, I'm Hungry!"*

As word spread, the project took on a life of its own. A Facebook page was set up—back when Facebook was still a baby—and suddenly, people all over the world were fundraising. There were bake sales in the UK, military personnel running for Chase, and even people riding bikes for donations. Our goal? $25,000.

Over 18 months, we held dozens of fundraisers, but two stood out. The first was the *Big Fat Gypsy Party*, where everyone dressed in outrageous outfits, and Chase, always the star, took the stage to sing with the band.

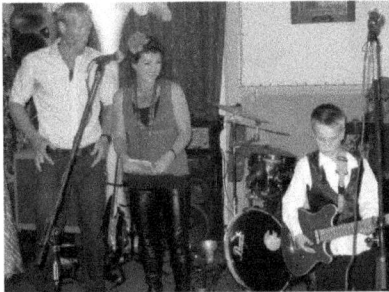

Then came the pinnacle: the *Gala Dinner with Helen Clark*, former Prime Minister and now a friend of Chase's, thanks to a previous encounter during the 2008 election campaign. She graciously agreed to be our guest speaker, and the event was shaping up to be the highlight of the entire project.

Of course, Chase had to get sick. Again.

At this point, we had perfected the art of "medical negotiations." Chase was transported from the hospital to the venue just long enough to shake Helen's hand, introduce her on stage with all the charm in the world, and then be promptly whisked back to his hospital bed before his temperature spiked again. Just another day in our world.

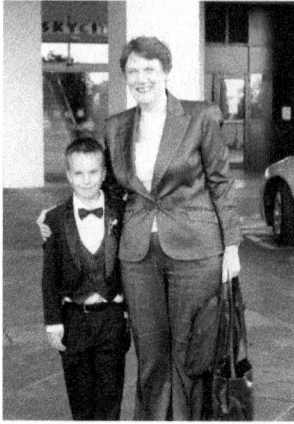

This ability to power through sickness wasn't new.

When Chase was four, we planned our first-ever family holiday to the Gold Coast. I should have known fate would throw a curveball. At midnight, the day before we flew, I realised he was sick.

Now, the rational parent might have said, *"We should cancel."*

But I was not a rational parent. I was a tired, stubborn, *desperate for a holiday* parent.

My reasoning? *"There are doctors in Australia, and I know the signs. A few days of antibiotics, and he'll be fine."*

So, we boarded the plane with Chase looking pale but still flashing his signature grin, which was usually enough to distract people from the fact that he was running a fever.

Everything was fine—until we started descending.

Chase turned to Steve and said the words no parent wants to hear at 30,000 feet: *"I need to burp."*

Translation? *"I'm about to redecorate the plane with my lunch."*

Steve, ever the hero, cupped his hands under Chase's mouth while I frantically searched for the sick bag. I was too late.

One second, Steve was a dad excited for this vacation. The next, he was covered in vomit, staring at me with the dead eyes of a man questioning all his life choices.

Ahh, the joys of parenting. If it worked for our trip to the Gold Coast – surely it New York would be fine, with perhaps just a little more preparation and a whole lot of insurance cover!

Despite the chaos, the fundraising, the hospital dashes, and the occasional airborne vomit incident, the project was a success. People from all over came together to make Chase's dream a reality.

And I, a woman who once couldn't ask for money without wanting to disappear into the floor, had somehow turned into a full-fledged fundraiser, hustling like a pro.

It was happening. Chase was going to New York.

Now, I just had to survive taking him there.

Chasing Life With CF

The dream was alive, the fund raising work going gangbusters .. life was busy. Sometimes I had to remind myself why we were doing this. This crazy late night events, this constant effort of talking with people, organising and connecting.. the 'Why' sometimes got lost in the energy.

Before Chase came into our lives, it feels like I had lived a whole other lifetime. A life filled with all-night parties, spontaneous road trips to nowhere, just me and the open road, music blasting, and the world feeling like it was full of endless possibilities. Relationships were simple, free of the worry that somehow, you'd be forced to choose between your own well-being and the well-being of someone you loved. You could sleep through the night without listening for every cough, every breath, every tiny shift in the rhythm of your child's chest. But that was before Chase.

Once CF arrived, our world, his world, became a blur of doctor's appointments, prescriptions, and an endless shuffle of bills that needed paying. All those carefree moments—gone in the blink of an eye. And yet, we wouldn't have it any other way. Chase's story became our story, and in a way, it was as though my own life hadn't truly started until he was born. It's a strange thing, really, how parents tend to forget the 'before.' We don't remember the carefree late-night talks with friends or the way our relationships once felt so effortlessly strong. We forget what it was like to live without the weight of the world on your shoulders. When your child is born with CF, your whole existence shifts. Every decision, every day, revolves around the disease in a way that makes everything else seem almost irrelevant.

I often laugh, albeit with a sombre edge, at how quickly we adapt to this new normal. People say it all the time—"You just adapt." But, you never really get used to it. The relentless barrage of hospital visits, the tests, the medications, the constant worry that the next set of results might show another setback, another complication. The thing about CF is that it's always there, lurking in the background, never quite letting you breathe easy.

For Chase, the liver complications were one of the first things we had to face. It's not uncommon for young children with CF to develop liver issues. The thick, sticky mucus that builds up in the lungs also blocks pathways throughout the body, including in the liver. As it becomes less efficient, the strain grows. We were told time and again that the liver could handle some of it, but there were moments, especially in those early years, when we wondered just how much more it could take. Every blood test, every scan, was another check on the list of things that were, or weren't, working. The liver numbers seemed like they had a life of their own, always fluctuating, always hinting at trouble. It was a constant worry, but one that we could only ride out as best we could, hopeful that Chase's resilience could keep pace.

And then there was his lung function. Oh, the lungs. They're the big one in CF—always the focus. But here's the kicker: they never go back to where they were. It's like climbing a mountain, only to slide down a little bit each time. We'd come in for a lung function test, and there would be a hopeful moment when the numbers were better than last time. But then, when we tested again, those numbers would dip a little lower. Always just a little less than before. It's like trying to hold onto a balloon that keeps slipping through your fingers. You can grab it again, but you know it's not quite as full as it once was.

And then there's the cough. The cough is relentless. Not because it's loud or constant, but because it's always there, lingering like an uninvited guest. It keeps you awake at night—not from the noise, but from the dread that creeps in with every wheeze, every fit of coughing. The fear that something else, something worse, might be lurking around the corner. We all know it. The slow, steady realisation that the disease is always progressing, always looking for new ways to push its boundaries. And in that moment, you're not just a parent—you're a full-time investigator, scanning for every clue, every symptom. Is there clubbing of the fingers? Bone brittleness? Kidney issues? Every time we had a new symptom to address, I found myself Googling the latest research, hoping that we'd find a way to stay one step ahead.

What never seemed to fail us, though, was the heart. The heart, that strange organ that keeps on beating even when everything else feels like it's falling apart. Chase's heart, much like his spirit, remains untouched by CF. I have no scientific evidence, no official reports to back it up, but I'm convinced that his heart is made of something strong—something unbreakable.

Maybe it's a twist of fate, or maybe it's something deeper, something more poetic. After all, Chase's heart has been tested, in ways none of us ever expected. Love interests came and went, breaking his heart, but each time, like a phoenix, it keeps pumping. No matter the pain, no matter the fear, it keeps moving forward.

And that's the thing about living with CF: it's a constant fight. But it's not a fight that Chase fights alone. We all fight it with him. It's a battle that doesn't ask permission, doesn't warn you when the next wave is coming. But you learn to stand tall in the face of it, because, despite it all, there's always that small glimmer of hope. The lung function tests, the liver tests, the bone scans—they may always be a little worse than before, but there's still life in those lungs, still strength in that heart.

Chase's story is my story now. It's the story of relentless courage, of a heart that never gives up, and a family that learns, again and again, how to hold on tight and keep moving forward. Sometimes the path forward takes sudden turns.... As we did in 2012.

"It's Over. (And, No, I Don't Mean 'The Sandwiches')"

Ending something as profoundly deep as a marriage is not easy. You don't wake up one morning and go 'Ok let's move on'.

Sometimes, you hit a point in life where everything feels like it's slowly spiralling into an emotional blender—only it's set to *puree* and you can't reach the off switch. For months—okay, years—I felt like I was running on fumes. Emotionally, I mean. The kind of fumes that you get when you've been living in a world of medical appointments, bills, and *not living*... really *living*. Sure, we existed. We were doing the thing we were supposed to do: wake up, drink coffee, go to work, manage a household, repeat. But somewhere in the abyss of daily tasks, I realised I had stopped really *living*. And I couldn't ignore it any longer.

Here's the thing: I've got a decent set of communication skills. I can talk circles around most people and make it sound like a TED Talk. I'm the type of person who can express my feelings so clearly that even the most complicated emotions look like a simple IKEA instruction manual. But when it came to this... *this*... communicating with Steve about the end of our marriage? Well, let's just say, I was the opposite of eloquent. I had all the right words in my head, but when I opened my mouth, it was like my tongue and brain were operating on different frequencies, sending out a scrambled signal.

So, one fateful afternoon, after months of internal wrestling and emotional disconnection, I just... blurted it out.

"It's over."

I know, I know. You probably expected something more graceful, like a heart-to-heart over dinner with a side of candlelight and tissues. Nope. Just... *"It's over."* Simple. Direct. But utterly shocking.

And, oh boy, the aftermath. What followed was three months of what I can only describe as an emotional rollercoaster... without any of the safety harnesses. It was like I'd suddenly stopped being in the marriage, emotionally speaking, and now had to catch up on the *physical* part. We were both still technically married, but I had already emotionally moved out. I was like a ghost in the house, walking around like Casper but with more passive-aggressive post-it notes stuck on the fridge.

The first few weeks were *loud*. Very loud. The type of loud where people might question if you've accidentally started a podcast about conflict resolution—except this one had *zero* resolution and a lot of shouting. Quiet arguments erupted into full-blown wars, with me making cutting remarks that I later regretted (as one does when you're in an emotional blender). I'm pretty sure Steve wasn't the biggest fan of my comments about how his "communication skills were as useful as a screen door on a submarine." But hey, it's all part of the process, right?

There were also moments of calm, as if we could *undo* the hurtful words we'd just thrown at each other. I kept hoping we could somehow shove all the nasty things back in their metaphorical box, never to be spoken of again, but nope. No box was big enough. The damage had been done, and I was resolute. I wanted us to *live*. And that, my friends, was non-negotiable.

And then, to make matters even more *delightful*, we had a New York trip still on the calendar. It was July, and the trip was scheduled for December. I had plenty of time to wrap my head around this, sort out the mess I'd created, and figure out what life actually looked like post-"it's over."

That's when I found the cottage. It was small. A kitchen no larger than a shoebox and was carpeted if you can believe that! It was cold—like *arctic* cold—but hey, small spaces are easier to heat, right? I didn't care. It had a treehouse, and that was all that mattered. The boys deserved somewhere they could call their own. Joshua was thrilled, Chase... well, Chase didn't even blink. He was too busy being Chase.

Moving in wasn't easy. There were tears and tantrums—mostly from me trying to fit an entire life into what was essentially a glorified shed. But it was ours. We had limited furniture, yes, but we were blessed by friends who delivered everything we needed. I'm talking sofas, bed frames, a single spoon (thank you, friends), and maybe, just maybe, some seriously questionable second-hand rugs. But it was a home now. It was a place where we could breathe, really breathe.

The first two weeks? No communication. Zero. Zilch. Nothing. I told the boys that I needed those two weeks for us. Just us. To find our new rhythm, our new reality. Joshua was confused at first, asking for his dad every two minutes, crying himself to sleep at night while my heart broke for him, but eventually, even he started adjusting.

And then there was Chase, who treated the whole thing like it was just another Tuesday. This kid, I swear—he could live through a hurricane and just keep humming his favourite tune. If anything, he was the glue that held it all together. There are days even now that I am thankful he doesn't live beyond the moment. He feels the hurt of the past I know. He feels it deep in his soul. His heart carries him through the hurt to the moments in the day that distract from the hurt.

The medical team wrapped themselves around us like we were in some kind of support group, knowing that, statistically speaking, divorce was a common side effect of chronic illness like CF. It wasn't surprising, but still, the whole thing felt like a weird, unspoken agreement between us all. You know, the *'Hey, we're here for you because you're probably going to need us after this whole marriage thing'* kind of support.

And so, life began. New home. New rules.

Chase was 11 and Joshua 4 – he would be 5 in 2013 and that became our future goal – Joshua going to school.

It was to be a *whole* new journey of emotional turmoil, self-discovery, and questionable interior decorating choices. It wasn't easy. It wasn't pretty. But we were living again. And for the first time in a long time, that felt like enough.

"Chase's Magical Christmas Adventure"

Despite a separation and the challenges associated with moving out of the family home, starting again we still had a dream to accomplish. Yes the dream...

It started with a dream. A dream that, as it turned out, was not just for Chase, but for all of us. A dream of Christmas in New York. A white Christmas, of course—because what is New York in winter without a little snow to make it feel like the movies? But this wasn't just any trip. No, this was *Chase's* dream adventure. We were going to visit all the iconic places from *Home Alone 2: Lost in New York*— because why not? If you're going to do New York, you do it properly.

But the adventure wasn't exactly as straightforward as it sounded. You see, planning a trip for Chase is always a little more complicated than booking flights and packing bags. It's an Olympic event of preparation. We were traveling with more medication than the pharmacy down the street, and every little detail was accounted for, right down to the backup inhalers, nebulizers, and enough antibiotics to fill a small suitcase. The one thing I *did* forget, however? My mother-in-law's Christmas gift—her fancy new nail clippers. But that's probably for the best because who really needs to get arrested at airport security before the trip even starts? It's the little things.

We made it through security with the usual mix of stress and careful smiles, and then it was finally time. We were going to New York. The plan was simple, right? Arrive, enjoy a white Christmas, see all the sights, and make magical memories. But somehow, in the middle of it all, the plan *changed*. The first twist came when, after some *last-minute negotiations* (and some seriously clever convincing), I managed to keep Joshua with his dad for Christmas. I'd thought about bringing him along, but after a brief emotional tug-of-war, we agreed it would be better for him to have a calmer holiday at home. It was a decision that stung a little—after all, it was Christmas, and I would miss him desperately—but I knew he'd be well cared for and have a great time.

Now, onto Chase. Everything is set; itinerary including hotels and connecting flights. First stop, unbeknown to Chase was LA. Well, he knew we were stopping in LA. What he didn't know was that we were staying in LA for a week before flying onto NY. His excitement for visiting NY and heading to Central Park or The Grand Plaza was evident. The adventure of a lifetime was becoming real.

The landing in LA began with a visit to the cockpit before disembarking with incredible support from the flight crew who were now in on the big secret! Helping keep the secret they told us that we would have to stay in LA due to weather in NY but not to worry everything was sorted.

Chase, none the wiser and more than tired after the 14hour flight simply went with the flow. My heart was bursting with excitement for him... and as we pulled into the carpark of the hotel in LA where the words DISNEYLAND were splattered everywhere.

Chase grabbed his carry bag and followed me to the check in desk. Even when the Concierge greeted us with 'Welcome to the Home of Disneyland" Chase didn't flinch. Then something in him shifted. His eye caught a glimpse of a flashing light. And almost if a lightbulb lit at exactly the same time somewhere in his far reaches of his brain - his eyes widened.

The word 'Disneyland' had made its way through. His eyes flitted to me full of questions... my simple nod was enough for all of the pieces come together. The secret nods and winks from the crew.

The whispers and closed-door meetings for fund raising. The hiding of the itinerary from him... Yes He realised where he was - The most magical place on earth.

His face lit up in a way that made me cry. All the hard work by so many had made this happen and they wouldn't be here to see it. Even his dad wouldn't be there to see the pure joy of his son. That made me sad. However, Disneyland is not a place for sad. The next week was a blur of rides, Disney characters of my own childhood, food, sore feet, more food, and Space Mountain Screams! Medieval dinners donated by a kindly sponsor, nights on the balcony watching the fireworks, afternoons lazing by the pool before dinner and the promise of more memory making the next day.

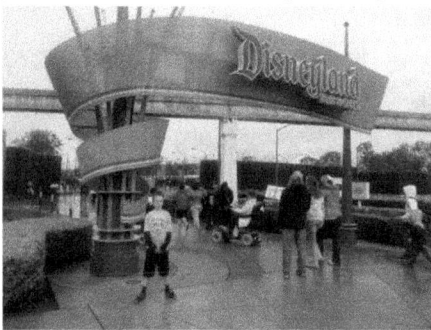

Yet NY still beckoned. Hurricane Sandy had swept through a few months earlier and we had heard the weather wasn't great. So as we spent the last days in LA buying souvenirs and gifts, my mind began to move to managing Chases health for the most important part of the adventure. He was already showing signs of tiredness. So there were a few extra 'rest' breaks during the fun filled days.

3 days before Christmas Day, we landed in Newark Airport - it was cold and grey. And in a typical NY Yellow Cab we were crossing the bridge into NY City! Chase was glued to the window breathing in

every sight of this wonderous city. My eyes continued to scan for any falter in Chase.

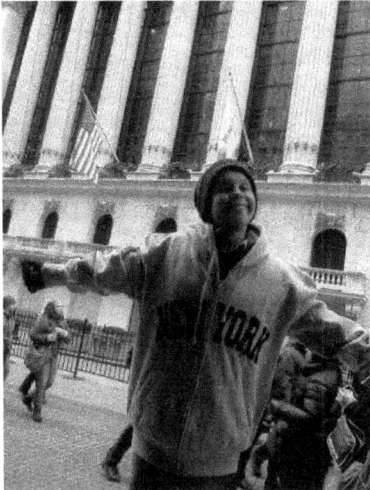

Any slight breathlessness or bout of coughing that would lead to him vomiting. He was always polite with it – he would always get to the bathroom in time. I have NO idea of how he learned that. When he was tiny – about 3yrs old he would be in the bathroom leant over the toilet heaving away, His legs shaking as I simply cradled him from behind holding him upright before passing him a cool cloth to wipe his face. I couldn't stop the damage, but I could support him in any way I was able. As he got older, I wasn't needed to hold him, I still give him a cool facecloth if needed.

New York - looking back, sometimes it feels like a lifetime ago. There have been more adventures since, but never one as big as this was.

We took a limousine ride to the most amazing toy shop in the city. It was like walking into a child's dream—every shelf stocked with the coolest, most bizarre toys you could imagine. We danced on the floor piano from the movie Big – the irony was not lost on me. Chase's eyes were wide with wonder as he walked from aisle to aisle, touching everything, trying to decide what he *needed* to bring home.

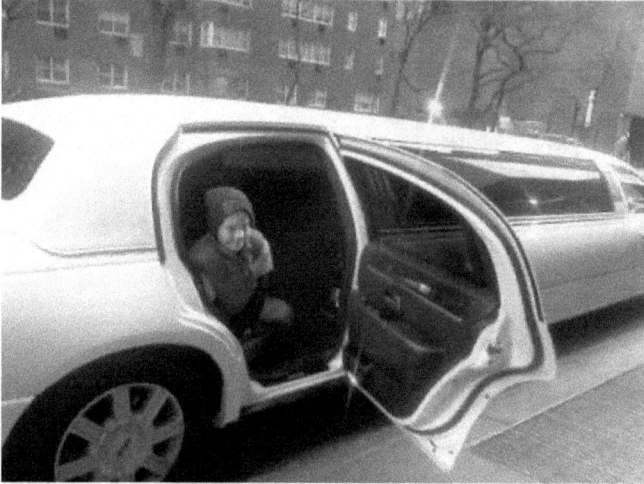

And then there was the ice skating in Central Park. If you've never seen it, you *should*—there's something incredibly magical about skating in the middle of Central Park, surrounded by the skyline and trees that are dusted with snow. Chase took to the ice like a natural, gliding around with a grace that was equal parts skill and sheer *joy*. It was the kind of moment that made you want to stop and breathe it all in, knowing that this was one of those memories that would be etched in both of our hearts forever.

A special moment for Chase, was when we went on a guided tour of the Metropolitan Museum of Art. As we walked through the galleries, he turned to me, wide-eyed, and said, "Mum, this is like *Night at the Museum*... for real." And he was right. The museum came alive in front of him. Each piece seemed to tell a story, and for once, it wasn't just about the disease or the constant worry—it was about art, history, and living in the moment.

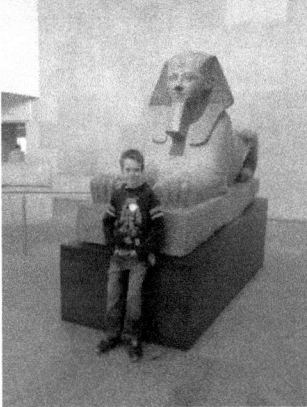

We ticked off all the must-see landmarks: the Empire State Building (which looked even more magnificent when we saw it lit up at night), the Statue of Liberty, and, of course, the ball drop on New Year's Eve. We watched the ball drop from the comfort of our hotel room, all cozy and warm, surrounded by those who, like us, were embracing the magic of the moment. Being in New York on New Year's Eve, without the crowds, felt surprisingly intimate and special.

We went to Ground Zero. There is an energy there that is hard to describe. For me, Ground Zero stood as a place of solemn reflection, resilience, and remembrance, a stark contrast to what we had seen on TV all those years ago when Chase was only a few days old. What we saw back then was the chaos, devastation, and overwhelming grief of September 11, 2001. The TV screen was full of the aftermath of the attacks, the site filled with smoke, rubble, and an eerie silence broken only by the sounds of emergency responders and the cries of those searching for loved ones. Now, years later, we stood in the same space, a space transformed into a memorial of honour and healing. The 9/11 Memorial pools, where the Twin Towers once stood, cascaded endlessly, symbolizing loss but also endurance as we both lightly swept our hands over the names of the lives lost. The sense of occasion was not lost on Chase, and he slowed down in that space. It was as if the butterfly had settled. It was a special moment for both of us.

Adventures from the hotel were a mix of carefully planned researched expeditions before completely random and spontaneous mission. A trip around the block to discover we were close to the Lincoln Center providing Chase with an unplanned overconfident tightrope walk around the edges of the Plazas fountain , arms outstretched for balance, sneakers squeaking on the wet stone, and a look on his face that said, *I am the master of this fountain...*Until a police officer blew his whistle telling Chase to get down!

Or the times we managed the 2min walk to Central Park for Chase to climb Umpire Rock while i relaxed for a few minutes. Or having had snow we had our first snowball fight - I won unfairly of course. Discovering the Central Zoo Park - the basis of the film Madagascar. Oh, we were both in heaven with all of the movie delights unfolding in front of us on a daily basis. And we only had days. But they were special days.

Of course we visited the iconic Home Alone - Lost in NY locations and were enthralled as we shouted at each other the scenes as they unfolded before us.

The Hudson Hotel - 58th Street NY was our base. Well, more of a haven, a dark sophisticated abode that was made for the funky at heart. For us it was a home - a small home, but home nonetheless.

The Deli on the corner provided my daily coffee and salad while Chase slept and rested safely ensconced in our room. And there were the staff.

The cherry on top was when we arrived at the Hudson Hotel. They had gone above and beyond to make our stay unforgettable. A Christmas tree was up in our room, with gifts just for Chase. I'm not sure how they knew, but it was the perfect touch. As if the city itself had wrapped its arms around us, making us feel as if we belonged there. That night, it snowed—a soft, perfect snowfall that covered the streets and made everything feel even more like a winter wonderland.

As we sat by the window, watching the snow fall on Christmas Day, I thought about how this trip—this incredible, unbelievable, once-in-a-lifetime adventure—had come together. Every moment, planned to perfection. Every detail considered. Medications packed. Room for gifts left. All because of the generosity of so many people— family, friends, strangers—who had worked together to make this dream a reality for Chase. And despite everything, despite the illness and the struggles, we were living. Truly living. I missed Joshua and that Christmas prayed I would never miss another Christmas without Joshua.

For me the NY adventure wasn't just a trip. It was a statement. A statement that we could do this—*we could live*—even in the face of challenges. And no matter what the future held, we would always have this adventure, this white Christmas, this magical journey to remind us of the power of hope, love, and community. And that, my friends, is the best kind of Christmas miracle there is.

"A New Normal, A New Horizon"

Coming back from New York was like waking up from a dream that was too beautiful to hold onto for long. We had experienced so much magic, so much wonder, and then reality came rushing back in, demanding its space. The apartment was quieter now, with no more laughter echoing through the rooms from surprise gifts or spontaneous ice-skating adventures. Instead, there was the hum of a new routine—one that was just starting to take shape but hadn't quite settled into place. We had to find our new normal, and it wasn't going to be as simple as slipping back into the old patterns we'd once known.

I was still working for myself, juggling projects, making ends meet. It wasn't easy, but somehow, we got by. There were days I'd wake up and wonder if it was all going to work out, but we always found a way. We had what we needed—maybe not everything we wanted, but we were making it work. Chase was adjusting to life after the trip. He'd returned to school, and while there was an undeniable sense of wonder and excitement in his eyes from everything we'd experienced, there was also the harsh reality of trying to fit in. For a young boy who was already *different*, trying to make new friends in a new school was no easy feat. He didn't have the luxury of just being "one of the crowd." CF didn't make him a "regular" kid, and sometimes that made things feel more challenging than they should have been.

I remember watching him at the school gates, trying to find a way into the social circles of his peers, and I could see how it affected him. It wasn't just the illness that made him different, it was the fact that he *knew* he was different. Kids can sense it. They know when someone stands apart, even if it's not immediately obvious why. But we got by, didn't we? We were learning how to navigate this new chapter, even if we didn't always have the answers. One step at a time.

Joshua, too, was getting ready for school. There was a lot of excitement in the house as we prepared for his first day—new backpack, lunchbox, the whole shebang. But with Joshua starting school, a whole new set of questions began to bubble up in my mind. It was a quiet realisation, something I hadn't fully faced until now: *What happens next?*

As I watched him get ready for a world of school, I couldn't help but wonder what the longer-term looked like for all of us. The idea of a "new normal" had already started to take shape, but I began to see that it might need to be bigger, different, more transformative. For months, I'd heard whispers of alternative medical treatments available in Australia—something about a different approach to CF. I had friends in Australia already, including Chase's Godmother, Shelly. She had always raved about the warmth and the drier climate, and I began to wonder if maybe, just maybe, the change could be exactly what Chase needed. The idea settled slowly into my mind, like a seed that had been planted and was now beginning to sprout.

The more I thought about it, the more it made sense. The weather would be better for Chase—drier air could potentially help with his lungs. There was the possibility of better treatments, more opportunities. And, above all, it felt like a place where we could *live*—not just exist, but truly build a life, with the community and support we needed, with a sense of freedom and opportunity for all of us.

But there was one big question that still loomed: *When?* & would Steve let us go. Joshua starting school had suddenly defined the timeline for me. If we were going to make this move, it had to be before he started. Once he started school, that was it—there'd be no turning back. We'd be tethered to the routine, to the life we had built here, and there would never be an easy time to upend it all.

So, like everything else we had done in life, the planning began. Steve funnily enough agreed with no argument at all. That felt surreal. And, of course, nothing about this was going to be simple. There was the logistics of moving across the Tasman, the practicalities of a whole new life. What do we take, what do we leave behind. Then there was the work for me and schools, healthcare for us as well as for Chase. Which CF clinic would we be attached to. I started researching everything. The team who had been with us from the moment Chase was diagnosed were beside us all the way – making the connections with the new hospital tam. Sharing details about Chase – his uniqueness and his CF related issues. Shelly and my other friends in Australia were more than supportive, but the reality of moving a family halfway around the world came with its own set of challenges.

But we were no strangers to challenges, were we?

Steve began to thaw a little. His visits with the boys were becoming more regular, and though things were still strained between us, there was a glimmer of hope that, with time, we could figure this out. The space between us was still palpable, but we were slowly learning how to coexist, to be parents, to support the boys in this new, fractured reality. There were moments of peace, brief but precious, when the boys would all be together, and we would pretend, just for a second, that things were normal again. It wasn't the fairy tale I'd once imagined, but it was enough. And sometimes, that's all you need.

And so, we began our new normal. It was simple, messy, and at times a bit overwhelming, but it was ours. Every day felt like we were just getting by—no more, no less. I would wake up in the morning with a million things to juggle, and at night I would fall asleep knowing we had made it through another day. There were days I thought we couldn't do it, days I wondered if I was making the right decision for all of us, but there were also days when I saw something in Chase's smile, in Joshua's excitement, that reminded me we were on the right path.

We were figuring it out. Slowly, surely, we were building a life. And as the idea of Australia started to take shape, it became clear to me that it was more than just a dream—it was a new beginning. For all of us.

As we walked into this new chapter, I wasn't sure what the future held, but I knew we had something that mattered most: we had each other, and that was a good enough foundation to start from.

And the new life begins

The last few days in our little cottage felt like a dream teetering on the edge of reality, each moment tinged with the duality of excitement and sorrow. Everything bound for the plane was meticulously packed, Chase's medications close at hand, Joshua's well-loved blankie safely tucked alongside him. The rest of our belongings—the things we could not bear to part with—were already secured in a container, waiting to board a ship bound for Australia, our new home.

We said goodbye to the team at the hospital. There were tears and cake as we said Thank you for being there for us every step of the way! When you live with an illness such as CF, people whom you would never generally meet become like family. People you rely on. People who gently but clearly tell you what's next. People who care deeply even. Don't ever let anyone say 'its just their job'. It is more than that, it is a vocation!

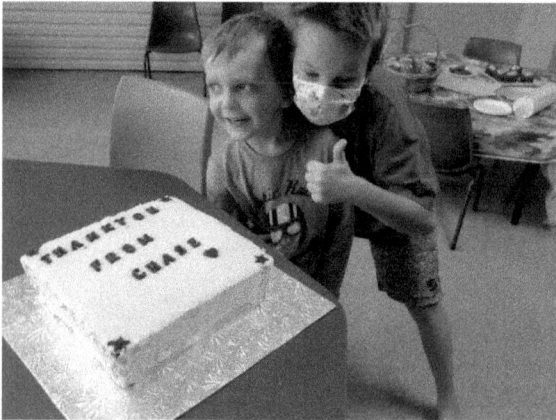

Two nights before our departure, I fell sick—a cruelly timed stomach bug that left me curled in pain, unable to move from the bed. I suggested, only half-joking, that I might not survive the night, and after some reluctant grumbling, Steve took the boys, giving me the solitude I needed to recover. For a fleeting moment, my dramatic claim felt almost justified as I lay there, fevered and miserable.

Despite the fever, I drifted through memories, each one a bittersweet echo of what we were leaving behind. The tiny backyard, just big enough for fireworks on special occasions, the night I was caught smoking on the porch, the sound of the boys' laughter at my guilty surprise. The ridiculous, frustrating, and ultimately hilarious moment when I installed Joshua's training wheels incorrectly, bolting the brackets upside down and leaving him to wobble precariously at a sharp angle—his determined little face confused but unfazed.

Monkey, my ever-loyal cat, was the last piece of the puzzle. She had been my constant through the years—before marriage, before children, through heartbreak and new beginnings. She had survived every move, every challenge, and even Chase's early childhood curiosity when he, in all his innocent logic, had tried to flush her down the toilet because he wanted a dog instead. After all, wasn't that where fish went when they were no longer needed?

On the final day, with the house locked and the car loaded, Monkey made a break for it, darting under the house just as I was ready to bundle her safely into the carrier. There was no other option—I stripped down to my underwear and crawled on my belly into the narrow, dust-filled space beneath the house. The rough ground scraped at my skin, cobwebs clung to my hair, but I pressed forward, my breath shallow in the musty darkness. At last, my fingers found her soft fur, and she let out an indignant yowl as I carefully dragged us both back into the light.

We delivered her safely to my mother's, where she would wait until we were settled enough to bring her over. The goodbye was heavier than expected, Monkey, ever stoic, sat in her carrier and watched me with those knowing eyes. It was a strange comfort, knowing that at least she wasn't going on this journey just yet.

And then came the hardest part: the farewell. We left the cottage behind; its walls still humming with the echoes of our lives and drove to the hotel for our final night before departure. When I picked up the boys after my night of sickness, Steve looked at me—just for a moment—with sadness in his eyes. He hadn't shown much emotion throughout the whole process, but in that instant, I felt it. Felt the weight of what we were leaving behind. He was saying goodbye, just as the boys were, and the promise of seeing them in the school holidays did little to fill the hollow pit in my chest.

We stood on the edge of something new, something vast and unknown. The adventure ahead was bright with possibility, but it was shadowed with the ache of parting. The cottage had been our safe harbor, a refuge in the storm of life. And now, we were setting sail into uncharted waters, hearts full of trepidation, hands grasping for the future.

Hide and Seek and Schoolyard Adventures

Moving to a new country with two kids and a new partner sounded like an adventure on paper. In reality? It was an Olympic-level event involving logistics, patience, and the kind of blind optimism usually reserved for people who jump out of planes for fun.

Our first hurdle? Our belongings, or rather, the complete lack of them. It was a strange phenomenon, living in a house that contained exactly one suitcase each, some borrowed furniture, and an overwhelming sense of "Where did I pack that again?" Waiting for our things to arrive became a full-blown game of Hide and Seek—with a twist.

"Mum! Where's my favourite shirt?"

"In a box. In the middle of the ocean. Somewhere."

"Muuuum! Where is my LEGO?"

"Also, in the ocean. Somewhere."

It was a fantastic parenting moment—giving the children an existential crisis about their beloved toys floating across the sea. Chase, ever the resourceful one, decided that if he couldn't play with his own things, he'd just find someone to hang out with – he did and soon we would have the neighbourhood kids kicking the footy around the front lawn. Joshua, my sweet, shy little one, found solace in playing "let's pretend we still have furniture" and would arrange pillows into elaborate makeshift forts. Honestly, I admired his creativity.

Luckily, we weren't doing this completely alone. Our friends opened their home to us for the first few weeks, which meant we had a soft landing as we found our feet. (And by "found our feet," I mean "figured out how not to get completely lost every time we stepped outside.") The city was enormous, filled with more people than our entire home country. It was like stepping into another world, one with actual public transport and endless streets that all seemed to look the same at first.

Amidst the chaos, getting the boys settled into school was the top priority. Joshua had just turned five two weeks before we flew out, which meant he barely scraped into the July school start. He was officially The Youngest. Most of his classmates were closer to six, making him the tiny, wide-eyed newcomer who clung to my leg with a vice grip of steel on that first day.

He was painfully shy and watching him step into that classroom felt like tossing a tiny, polite deer into a field of confident, experienced schoolyard wolves. But he persevered. Slowly, steadily, he found his rhythm. And, as I would later learn, became a teacher's favourite for his quiet smiles and impeccable manners.

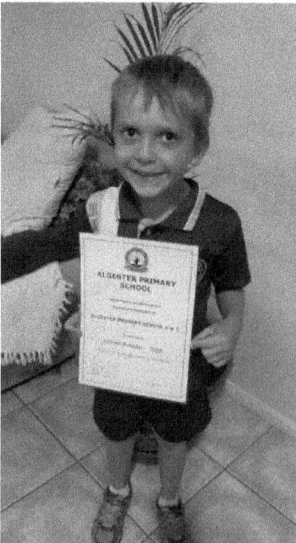

Meanwhile, I was navigating my own social jungle. Somewhere in this new land, I was about to meet a person who would change our lives—a soon-to-be best friend who would not only embrace my boys but also save my sanity by stepping in for before-and-after school care. As fate would have it, she was just as much a gift to me as she was to them, and with her help, I found a job, a routine, and a little piece of stability in the chaos.

And then there was Wayne.

Wayne, who had known me since I was 18. Who had been there in the background for years, cheering us on. And now? Now he was right in the thick of it, learning firsthand what it was like to be part of this ever-moving, ever-chaotic family. The learning curve was steep—for all of us.

"Did Chase just put his tablets in the letterbox?"

"Yes."

"...Why?"

"Because he doesn't want to take them."

"...Right."

Wayne took it all in stride (mostly). He had seen the challenges but living them was an entirely different experience. Still, we navigated it together, making up the rules as we went.

Six weeks in, and we finally had a place of our own. A rental close to the school, close to new routines, and close to feeling like we had our feet under us. The city still felt enormous, the roads still confusing, but we were doing it. We were building something new.

And best of all? Our belongings finally arrived. It was like Christmas morning, only with more panicked box-cutting and emotional reunions with previously lost stuffed animals. We had survived the first chapter of our new life.

What could possibly go wrong next?

The call that acknowledged the challenge

One week. That's all it took for the school to ring me about Chase.

Now, normally, when a school rings that early into a term, it's either because your child has set something on fire (accidental or otherwise) or has managed to convince their classmates that the principal is an undercover spy. So, when my phone lit up with the school's number, I braced myself.

"Hello, is this Chase's mum?"

"Yes... is he okay?"

"Oh, he's fine! We just wanted to discuss some learning difficulties we've noticed."

I could have cried. No—actually, I could have sung Hallelujah at the top of my lungs in the middle of the street. Finally! Someone saw what I had been seeing! Someone wasn't just giving me the standard, "He'll catch up." No, they were saying, "WOOOOO, we need to help him NOW or he'll NEVER catch up!"

Within days, there were referrals flying left and right—to learning specialists, educational psychologists, support teachers—more professionals than I had ever seen involved in Chase's life outside of a hospital. It was surreal. Up until now, every expert we had dealt with had been focused on his health, his Cystic Fibrosis. His lungs, his digestive system, his treatments, his hospital visits. But now? Now people were zeroing in on his brain, and for the first time, it wasn't just me wondering, "If his brain worked better, would his CF be better managed too?"

Of course, amidst all this sudden academic intervention, we still hadn't even had our first CF clinic. That felt weird. It was as if Chase had been rebranded overnight. No longer "Chase, the kid with CF," but "Chase, the kid who learns differently." It was almost a relief. Almost.

By the end of the week, I had so many meetings booked that I felt like Chase had somehow been cast as the main character in an elaborate, multi-agency crossover event. But, for the first time, I wasn't fighting to be heard. The system had seen him. And that, in itself, was a small miracle.

Primary school would go on to throw challenges at us that we hadn't anticipated such as exclusion. I had had to argue Chases case with a teacher that Chase deserved to go on school camp like all the other children. I shouldn't matter than he had a few extra body parts or needed constant medication. I was not about to let him be excluded. Her argument was that they didn't have enough staff to support Chases medication regime of physio and pills. It was 3 days – 2 nights. I said then we wont worry about physio. Let's just ensure he has his tablets. He will survive, he has managed to get to this point.

That was a fight we won!

Chase, the Mini Doctor

Children with Cystic Fibrosis spend so much time in hospitals that, by the time they reach school age, they could probably pass a medical exam with flying colours. Chase was no exception. He could navigate a hospital better than most interns and was more than happy to educate any unsuspecting medical students on the wonders of CF.

"Do you know why my mucus is thick? It's science."

Cue nervous nodding from the trainee doctors while Chase launched into an enthusiastic (and slightly gross) explanation about mucus, but his way "mum says its like wallpaper paste whatever that is here do you want to look as he would try to cough up some gunk for the unsuspecting doctor".

He also had two "bonus" body parts—his mickey button and his portacath. His veins had been useless since birth, a fact I knew all too well from his first hospital visit at four weeks old when no one could get a needle in. It never changed. By age three, he had a portacath put in, and from that moment on, he was basically a cyborg. In New Zealand, it needed flushing every month. In Australia? Every six weeks... sometimes longer. Each extra week made me stress that it might get blocked. Chase, on the other hand, simply saw it as another fun fact to add to his ever-growing medical knowledge vault.

"Mum, if I ever need a job, I could be a doctor!"

Honestly? He wasn't wrong except he was – his brain capacity would now be the additional hurdle to his CF world.

Cystic Fibrosis doesn't just affect the lungs—it blocks all sorts of vital functions, including digestion. This means many kids with CF struggle to absorb nutrients, leading to the classic CF look: small, skinny, and paler than a vampire at a sunscreen convention. Chase fit the mould perfectly.

By the time he was 12, we knew puberty was looming, and with it, his one shot at a decent growth spurt. This was our moment. We had to get calories into him at all costs. We entered the world of calorie stacking double cream, extra butter, high-fat everything. If a meal didn't have the calorie count of an entire football team's lunch, it wasn't good enough.

But Chase, living in a world of tanned, buff, beach-loving Australian kids, had no desire to bulk up. While other boys ran shirtless across the sand, looking like junior lifeguards in training, Chase was the kid who resembled a Victorian ghost child who might whisper warnings about a haunted attic.

"Maybe I'll just stay small," he once said, sipping his high-calorie milkshake laced with coconut oil while side-eyeing a particularly hefty 13-year-old.

"Or," I countered, "maybe you'll drink that shake and we'll make sure you don't get blown away in a strong breeze."

The growth spurt game was on, and we were playing to win.

We didn't know how badly we would lose this game.

If we had known, we might have taken a different path. One where I didn't work. One where I could homeschool him and keep him still so the calories didn't burn off. Where I could provide a steady stream of food continuously all day without fear it would end up in the bin. Or be there to ensure every tablet was taken.

Chase in his own finite wisdom chose his own path. We could not force feed him. And while I could tempt him with all manner of delights, with food being such a focus of his health for all these years – food just wasn't of interest to him. It was my interest, my passion. And frankly helped develop my cooking skills. We won't mention my baking skills – that have never evolved beyond a passable pancake! When your seven-year-old begs their teacher NOT to allow you to make a cake for the school fete you know your skills or lack thereof are well and truly understood!

So, puberty hits, Chase is moving to high school, and still his weight remains pitifully low. And amongst all these challenges we embarked on another drug trial all in the name of the CF Cause and finding a cure.

The Wild, Wacky, and Occasionally Effective Quest to Cure Cystic Fibrosis

If history has taught us anything, it's that humans will throw just about anything at an illness to see if it sticks. Cystic fibrosis (CF) is no exception. Over the years, we've seen everything from questionable herbal remedies to cutting-edge genetic wizardry to outsmart this stubborn disease. It's been a journey—sometimes frustrating, sometimes absurd, but ultimately one that's led to some incredible breakthroughs. I did so much research in the early years on my quest to save Chase. I discovered that with a disease like CF, inherited (not caught) and with so few people having it, doesn't make for great strides in medical breakthroughs. The research money outweighs the benefits... sounds harsh doesn't it!?

A simplistic way I saw this was that if you have 10 people with a disease that is going to take $5million dollars to research a cure, and then you have 5 thousand people with an illness you are going to put the $5million into to the area with the biggest positive outcome – in the marketing world, you are going to stack that ROI as much as you can! When Chase was born there were less than 350 people living with CF in NZ with a population of 3.1million people. That's less than .015% of people. Now consider the cancer statistics according to a study from Otago University 5.1% of New Zealanders lived with some form of cancer.

Making tough decisions with limited funding has always meant inherited diseases like CF affecting fewer people despite having what was then a certain fatal outcome wasn't a decision I would like to have been making.

Let's be frank, CF has been around for centuries, but for most of that time, nobody had a clue what it was. Back in the day, babies with salty skin were thought to be cursed—or, in some medieval circles, marked for an early demise. By the early 20th century, doctors finally started connecting the dots, but there was just one tiny problem: there was no actual treatment. If you had CF, you basically got a pat on the back, some vague dietary advice, and a "good luck, kid."

Then came the era of creative solutions. Some early physicians prescribed special diets packed with extra calories, believing that sheer caloric force could overpower the disease. (Spoiler alert: It did not.) Others encouraged "fresh air therapy," which was essentially just sending kids outside and hoping for the best. And then, of course, there were the obligatory snake oil salesmen peddling miracle elixirs made from who-knows-what.

By the mid-20th century, CF research started getting serious. Scientists figured out that thick, sticky mucus was the real villain in this story, clogging up lungs and digestive tracts. But what to do about it?

Enter: percussion therapy. If you grew up with CF in the 1950s or '60s even 70s in NZ, there's a good chance you spent a lot of time being smacked around, lovingly, of course. Chest physiotherapy (CPT) became a standard treatment, where a family member or therapist would thump on a patient's back and chest to loosen mucus. It was basically the medical equivalent of shaking a sauce bottle, and while it wasn't perfect, it helped.

At the same time, doctors discovered that adding extra salt to the diet could be beneficial. Since CF patients lost too much salt through their sweat, boosting intake was an easy (if unglamorous) fix.

Imagine being told to eat more potato chips for your health. Not the worst prescription.

By the time the '80s rolled around, CF treatment was looking a little more sophisticated. Inhaled medications helped open airways, while digestive enzymes finally allowed patients to absorb nutrients properly instead of, well, just watching them pass right through.

Then, in 1989, the game changed completely. Scientists discovered the actual genetic mutation responsible for CF: a faulty CFTR gene. This was like unlocking the boss level of the disease—suddenly, we knew what we were fighting. Researchers now had a target, and the race for truly effective treatments kicked into high gear.

The early 2000s saw the rise of CFTR modulators, drugs that helped correct the underlying problem instead of just managing symptoms. This wouldn't hit New Zealand though for nearly another 15years.

Kalydeco was the first of these, hitting the market in 2012. It was a miracle for some, but it only worked on a small percentage of CF patients with a particular mutation. Next came Orkambi. I have a certain amount of pride knowing Chase was part of the trial for Orkambi here in Australia. Participating in a drug trial or any medical trial takes commitment and dedication. We had been doing it all of Chase's life. So when we landed in Australia within two months we had been asked if we would participate in what would be the first of two trials.

The first - a trial on whether giving a baby anaesthetics had an effect on their psychological or intellectual outcomes. I have so many questions about this still to be answered, that perhaps is another book!

The second, was the Orkambi Drug Trial. Two arms – placebo and the actual drug. Monthly check-ups, constant blood taking to measure liver function. Eyes checked at the beginning of the trial, bone density and all manner of measurements taken.

Here we were, still settling into our new lives, me working, Wayne taking care of us all and the boys in school. Every month I was needing to juggle taking time off to get Chase to clinic for evaluation. It wasn't long, perhaps 12months in when the strain began to take a toll. With all the issues at school and Chases integration into a mainstream school that identified his learning challenges, me trying to work fulltime travelling 2 hours a day, needing to support Joshua and a household... it all got a bit much. Chase asked to stop. He wanted to be normal.

He said the words 'Mum I want to be normal!'

We stopped. We withdrew from the drug trial. For me it was heartbreaking, knowing he potentially was stopping taking a drug that might in fact be saving his life. However I understood, I was tired too. And frankly if I was tired, I knew he must have been exhausted beyond belief.

I argued with myself that we hadn't seen a lot of difference, and the difference id seen at the beginning was possibly just in my head. The weight was still an issue. His lung function while it hadn't declined, hadn't improved. And his liver was still dodgy. The argument about how much time off work and school we were both having was a lot. No matter how much I used my annual leave or sick days, the realisation was that it was too much. We weren't living... and that was the kicker... I had left a marriage because we weren't living – and here I was doing it again!

So yes, we stopped participating in the Orkambi Drug Trial, it was only many years later that I found out we were in fact on the placebo.

But like all things, the show must go on and the drug trial continued without us with updates in science leading to Symdeko, which helped more people but still weren't the universal fix that everyone was hoping for.

Then, in 2019, Trikafta burst onto the scene like a medical rock star. This three-drug combo (elexacaftor, tezacaftor, and ivacaftor) changed everything. Unlike its predecessors, Trikafta worked for about 90% of CF patients, making it the closest thing to a cure that we've ever seen.

Patients who had spent their lives struggling to breathe suddenly found themselves, well, breathing. It was like someone had lifted a two-ton weight off their chests, because, in a way, they had.

Trikafta is incredible, but it's not the end of the road. Scientists are already looking beyond modulators, exploring gene therapy and even CRISPR technology to potentially fix the CFTR mutation permanently.

Being in Australia and NOT New Zealand meant we got access to Trikafta very early on. And it only cost us $38 a month. Soon Chase would only be paying $6, but that's another chapter...

For now, though, we can take a moment to appreciate how far we've come, from medieval superstitions to a drug that lets people with CF live longer, healthier lives. And if history has taught us anything, it's that the next breakthrough is always just around the corner.

High School Raises The Stakes.

Chase had made it this far in life with a smile, a giggle or completely unmemorable joke. And now he was off to high school. Noting that I am an organiser (Wayne would suggest control freak!) there had been early discussions about which high school. We had to consider travel, support options and closeness to hospital. And in my mind, it had to be mainstream so he would be 'normal' and he would thrive!

I thought I was prepared. I really did.

New uniforms? Bought. School supplies? Labelled. Bus pass? Secured in a special pouch with a backup in my wallet.

Chase, however, was *not* prepared.

Day one of high school arrived like a tsunami. Chase's first challenge? The bus. The simple act of catching a bus became a saga worthy of its own documentary. First, he lost his bus pass. Not just once, but repeatedly, as though it had sprouted legs and wandered off the moment it entered his possession. On the occasions he *did* manage to keep hold of it, he'd forget to tap off, leaving me to discover horrifying travel bills that suggested he'd been commuting to another state.

Then came the overwhelming reality of *high school structure.*

Moving between classes? Utter chaos. Taking the right books to each lesson? A myth. Taking *any* book to class? An Olympic-level achievement.

By week one, Chase had already lost his brand-new $89 school jersey, which I assume vanished into the void where lost socks and Tupperware lids reside. By week four, the $75 math book—a brick-sized monstrosity heavier than Chase himself—had also disappeared into the abyss. I had my suspicions that some of his possessions were being sacrificed to an alternate dimension, but there was no time to investigate; I was too busy retrieving detention slips from his schoolbag.

The first term flew by in a haze of misplaced belongings and missed bus taps. Then, term two arrived, and with it—suspension number one. The crime? Personal space violations. Not violent, not aggressive, just... *too close*. Chase's definition of "appropriate proximity" did not align with mainstream society's. He simply enjoyed existing within the breathing zones of others. Apparently, this was not ideal.

Suspension number two? Even more ridiculous. Chase, in a moment of grand defiance, *declared* that he was leaving the school grounds. Did he leave? No. Did he fully intend to leave? Not particularly. But the *threat* of leaving was enough to earn him a one-way ticket to another 'family consultation' with the bald-headed deputy principal.

Ah, the deputy principal. A man who had already decided Chase's fate before we even sat down. I could feel it in the way he looked at me, in the condescending tone he chose at exactly the wrong moment. So, I asked him, had he in fact read the introduction document about Chase and his unique mannerisms. He hadn't. I suggested had he taken the two-minutes it would have taken he might have been able to deal with this differently. How a suspension didn't provide incentive to change, losing a privilege such as sports might. How expecting a young person with an IQ of just on 70 could be expected to navigate a complex system and succeed with little support was not OK surely... But looking at him sitting back in the chair arms folded glaring at me, I *knew* his mind was made up. And that's when it hit me—mainstream school was not for Chase, and Chase was not for mainstream school. I work within the mainstream school system now. I can tell you; it hasn't changed.

However, for us, it did change, we needed something different. Something that didn't see Chase's quirks as crimes. And so, the search began.

Enter: *The Special School.*

A place that welcomed us, portacaths, Mickey buttons, and my frazzled, slightly unhinged mum-energy included. A place that saw Chase for who he was: a hilarious, unique, *occasionally forgetful* kid with a bus pass vendetta. Chase left the battlefield of mainstream education behind, and for the first time, high school seemed... possible. Or at least, significantly less of a horror movie.

Chases first day, I had to be at work as I had used all my leave allocation, so Wayne took him. Apparently, Chase was met with a huge sloppy kiss from a fellow student as a welcome. Chase for once in his life was gobsmacked!

Chase made friends fast, teachers, other parents and students as well. The high gated school might have looked intimidating, but it was far from it. The staff were amazing and probably had to deal with far more than that balding deputy principal ever could, but they did it with laughter and smiles.

There were challenges of course.

Like the time Chase hit a stand in teacher. The teacher had pulled Chase back on the sideline from a game telling him that others had to play, and he could wait. With one of Chases only abilities – his ability to play sport, Chase felt the full force of unfairness hit him and he hit back. Chase was also the Schools Sports Captain and was often found helping other students, young people in wheelchairs or with disabilities creating significant challenges. He would help them catch or throw a ball. Chase believed it was his right to be on the field helping his peers, the stand in teacher wasn't aware. It was a classic miscommunication moment.

Kicking a teacher however was not appropriate of course. The Principal, a man I will forever hold close in my heart called me to tell me what had gone down. Chase was suspended and not allowed to play sport for a week. It was enough for Chase to fully understand the error. He would go onto helping at the next door mainstream high school with the HPE team setting up sports equipment. In the future he would become a rugby league referee. He was sports mad! Here he is in yellow, sometimes all we could look for was the splash of yellow as Chase was more often smaller than the players and hard to see!

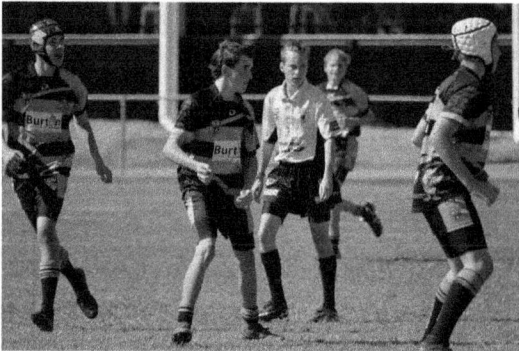

This school enabled us to have a few medical procedures done at school! Port flushes, physio, some OT when needed. It reduced the hospital visits. Teaching staff helped us when we needed cognitive assessments done to determine chases actual abilities. They provided the balance to my somewhat rosy coloured glasses viewpoint. No, he did not take his tablets unless reminded. Yes, he struggled to focus for any normal length of time. Yes, he needed constant reminding to do things that he did every day. Yes, he was great with people, but only in a very superficial way. Conversations were flighty and nonsensical. Guidance was needed constantly. His CF became a little less visible in this new education world of sickness and disability. But it was ours and we embraced it.

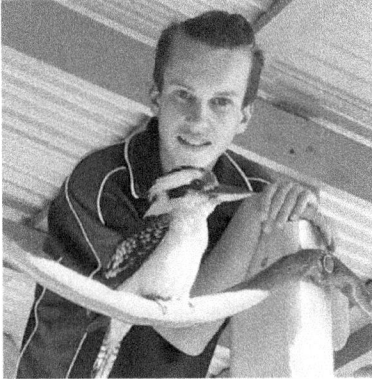

I vividly remember Chase being in the School Play. He was the lead and he studied so hard even teaching staff got worried. They wanted him to enjoy it. Somehow Chase knew he was on show and wanted it to be the best he could be. He nailed it for that performance. My heart soars when I think of him now strutting his stuff as the wolf in a 1950s version of Little Red Riding Hood! He shone like I had never seen – he had made it in high school!

He was School Captain, had his first serious girlfriend going to his formal twice... yes he got held back another year which was fabulous because he wasn't ready for the world, and the world wasn't ready for him... in some ways it still isn't. He even represented his school and New Zealand in a video for ANZAC day. He was constantly making me proud.

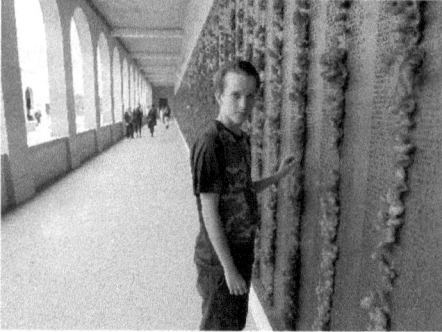

So high school turned out to be a magical time for Chase. CF took a back seat; education took the lead and we all survived. Life was about to throw one more major medical hurdle at us which none of us could have prepared for. However, for now, life was settled.

Footnote: When the mainstream school sent us a bill for the math book, I sent it back telling them politely to take me to court!

2018 – The Year Chase Almost Died (But Didn't, Because He's Stubborn)

2017 had been a year of triumph! Having got married in late 2016, Wayne and I had then realised another milestone and built our dream home brick by brick, mortgage by mortgage and moved in. It was ours. It was perfect. Chase was still able to remain at the special school with a bus collecting him from the front gate each day and delivering him back safely. We had a fabulous community and life was looking good. Joshua had settled quickly into a new school and was quietly making new friends. All was good with the world.

And then, because life enjoys a bit of dramatic irony, I quit my job.

Why? Well, my charmingly unethical boss asked me to do something illegal. When he threw out the classic "I pay you, so you do what I ask," I responded with, "You don't pay me enough, and from here on out, you don't pay me at all." I gracefully (read: dramatically) placed my keys on his desk, turned on my heel, and marched out the door while his bean-counting accountant watched in stunned silence. It was November. I had no job. Christmas was going to be... frugal.

When I broke the news to my husband, expecting at least a little panic, he just said, "Good on ya, girl. About time!" That man could make me feel better about an asteroid strike.

Christmas was quiet but not catastrophic. The boys were flying off to New Zealand to spend two weeks with their dad after Christmas. Perfect timing, because I had miraculously landed a new job starting in January. I would finally get to experience our house as a peaceful, child-free haven.

I had visions of quiet mornings with coffee, long baths, and spontaneous naps. I could finally breathe without the constant worry of "Has Chase taken his meds?" "Is Chase annoying his brother?" (Spoiler: He was. Always.)

And for a brief, shining moment, life was idyllic.

Then came Friday.

Just days into my new job, my phone rang. It was a private number.

Now, let's rewind 12 hours.

My phone had rung in the middle of the night on the Thursday. Half-asleep, I assumed it was my husband calling from work. Nope. It was the boys' dad.

"Chase has been vomiting for a few hours," he said. "Do you know if his liver results have been normal?"

Sleepy-brained me nodded (which is useless on the phone) and mumbled, "Yeah, they're normal."

Then I rolled over and went back to sleep.

In my defence, it was almost midnight my time, which meant it was 3 AM their time. Who takes a kid to the doctor at 3 AM unless that doctor is in an emergency room? I should have connected the dots, but I didn't. Instead, I woke up, sent a casual "How's Chase?" text in the morning, got no reply, and went about my day like a blissfully ignorant fool.

Cue: The Friday Phone Call.

On the other end was Chase's doctor from Brisbane. The conversation began with, "Have you booked a flight yet?"

That got my attention.

She then kindly suggested I sit down and proceeded to inform me that Chase was in the ICU. His liver and kidneys were shutting down. He had a rare, life-threatening condition called Haemolytic Uremic Syndrome (HUS).

Haemolytic Uremic Syndrome (HUS) is like the ultimate uninvited guest, it crashes into your body, causes absolute chaos, and leaves a mess for your kidneys to clean up. This condition typically happens when tiny blood vessels become inflamed and clogged with clots, leading to low red blood cell counts (haemolytic anaemia), low platelets (thrombocytopenia), and, worst of all, kidney failure. The most common culprit?

A nasty strain of E. coli, often picked up from contaminated food or water, though other infections, certain medications, and even autoimmune conditions can trigger it. HUS can range from a temporary nightmare with full recovery to a long-term battle involving dialysis or even a kidney transplant. Kids are the usual targets, but adults aren't off the hook. While treatment varies, ranging from IV fluids and blood transfusions to plasma exchange early diagnosis and supportive care are key to preventing long-term damage.

In short, it's a rare but serious condition that reminds us all to wash our hands, cook our burgers properly, and respect just how delicate our internal plumbing really is.

And it had nothing to do with his Cystic Fibrosis because clearly, one fatal disease wasn't dramatic enough for him. No, he had to go for the bonus round.

My heart dropped. I was two flights away, one three-hour flight and another one-hour connecting flight. Plus, I was already too late for the last flight of the day.

Cue: Panic Mode.

The next 24 hours were the longest of my life. I prayed, I screamed, I cried, and I experienced a level of stress normally reserved for hostage situations. But I had no choice but to wait.

Twenty-eight hours later, I finally arrived. I was met at the airport by my younger son, Joshua, and their dad. Joshua ran to me and simply said, "You're here!"

That was all it took to snap me out of my internal meltdown. I was here. Now, I had to focus.

When I walked into Chase's hospital room, I nearly collapsed. He looked terrible, yellow, swollen, and covered in tiny blood pinpricks. His eyes were bleeding. BLEEDING. Like something out of a horror movie.

But when he saw me, he smiled.

And in that moment, I knew he was going to be okay.

For the next three days, I stayed by his bedside, working with the medical team to explain what his "normal" looked like. I even brought a giant poster from his 16th birthday to show the doctors that, no, he was not supposed to look like an overinflated balloon.

The doctors warned that he'd be in the hospital for a long time. His body rejected antibiotics, feeding tubes made things worse, and every minor treatment seemed to backfire. And yet, this stubborn kid fought through it.

We played endless games of cards between naps, carefully managing his IV fluids to avoid overloading his fragile body. I watched in awe as he slowly but surely started improving.

By day three, he was stable. Not out of the woods, but stable.

And then I did the unthinkable, I left.

I know, I know. What kind of monster mother abandons her child in the hospital? A mother who just started a new job and needed to keep it.

His father wasn't thrilled with my "selfishness," but Chase was past the worst of it. My boss had already been kind enough to let me disappear for an emergency, and I couldn't push my luck.

So, I flew home, spent the next week pretending to function like a normal human, and counted down the days until my boys returned.

Ten days later, I met them at the airport with the biggest hugs imaginable.

Chase had survived. Because, of course, he did. The world wasn't done dealing with his particular brand of chaos yet.

Chase Flies the Coop (and Lands in a Lockdown)

Eighteen years. Eighteen years of school runs, misplaced belongings, and medical appointments. Eighteen years of making sure Chase had what he needed before he even knew he needed it. And now, finally, we had arrived at the moment I had been both anticipating and dreading in equal measure: *Chase was leaving school*.

Unlike many of his peers in mainstream, Chase had stayed for an extra year, soaking up the last remnants of structured education like a sponge that only absorbs half of what it's meant to. In that time, he had even managed to land a part-time job at McDonald's. Well, "job" might be a strong word—his shifts were so sporadic they could've been scheduled by a malfunctioning Magic 8 Ball. It quickly became apparent that McDonald's had a strong financial preference for hiring 17-year-olds who cost them less per hour. Still, the experience was something.

More consistent was his work as a rugby league referee. It paid a little, enough to keep him in weekend snacks and the occasional impulse purchase.

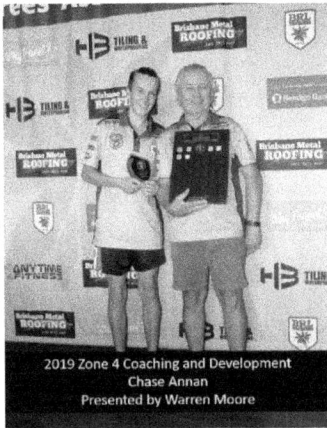

2019 Zone 4 Coaching and Development
Chase Annan
Presented by Warren Moore

But let's be real, it wasn't going to cover rent, groceries, or, heaven forbid, *bills*. And so, the looming question presented itself: *What next?*

Chase had already had a trial run at leaving home, though I'm not sure either of us intended it that way. One day, during a particularly heated argument, I told him to get out.

I meant for the *day*.

Chase took it as a permanent eviction notice.

With impressive speed, he packed his bags, caught a bus, and left. Just like that. Poof. Gone.

It wasn't until later that I realised he had found refuge at his girlfriend's parents' house. My first reaction was shock: *He actually followed through?* My second reaction? *Well, at least I taught him how to navigate public transport.*

He stayed away for months. In that time, he got a crash course in the realities of living under someone else's roof. House rules were not flexible guidelines; they were *rules*. Contributing to household chores was *not* optional. And as it turns out, despite his frequent attempts to pretend otherwise, *food does not magically replenish itself.*

Eventually, he returned, slightly wiser, slightly more appreciative of the world I had constructed for him. But that return was temporary. We both knew it. It was time to start thinking about something more permanent.

The thing about raising a child with significant medical needs is that, no matter how independent they seem, there's always that nagging fear: *Will they be okay without me?* For 18 years, I had been the one making sure he had his medications, filling scripts before they ran out, stocking the fridge and pantry with foods that worked for his health.

And now, I had to trust that all those years of preparation had actually prepared him.

I reminded myself of the mantra I had clung to since he was little: *I am raising him to live his life, not mine.* This was the goal all along. This was what all the lessons, the arguments, the reminders, and the structured chaos had been leading up to.

So, with equal parts excitement and terror, we signed a lease. Well, *I* signed as guarantor, because, let's be real, no landlord in their right mind was going to take an 18-year-old with McDonald's pocket money as their sole tenant. But still, the place was *his*. Chase had a flat.

And then, because the universe has an impeccable sense of timing, *the entire city went into COVID lockdown the very next day.*

Let's take a moment to appreciate the absurdity of the situation. My son, who had spent his entire life in an environment where everything was done for him *just enough* to keep him on track, was now fully independent.

In a lockdown.

On day one, he called me.

"Do I need to wash my clothes every day?"

Oh, dear Lord.

It became clear that, despite my best efforts, I had *not* covered every single aspect of independent living in my teachings. Chase's flat quickly became its own ecosystem, an experiment in what happens when an 18-year-old is left to his own devices during a global crisis.

Groceries were an issue. He had the skills to shop but *not* the patience to plan meals. He survived the first two weeks because I drove like a woman possessed daring any policeman to stop me – Chase was considered vulnerable, and I was allowed to travel for that reason only... I arrived armed with enough food to get him through the next few days. With a tiny fridge it was a challenge, but I would be back every day with replenishing stocks. Chase had casual work at the same place I was so I bought breakfast every morning and lunch so I knew he had two decent meals a day. Once lockdown hit, it was different. I didn't have eyes on him other than via Facebook. And he wasn't going to show me his entire space..

Housekeeping? A mixed bag. He wasn't *dirty*, but he also wasn't *diligent*. Dishes stacked up until they became a pressing issue. Laundry happened in unpredictable bursts of enthusiasm.

Medication? That was my biggest fear. For years, I had been the one keeping track of prescriptions, ensuring he never ran out of what he needed. Now, that responsibility fell squarely on his shoulders. It took a few close calls (and more than a few reminder texts), but he managed. He learned.

And slowly but surely, he adapted.

The lockdown stretched on, but so did Chase's ability to function independently. He would spend a long time soaking in a hot bath in his flat. Once lockdown lifted, he was back working and still refereeing.

He even started planning ahead—a shocking development for a boy who once considered "thinking about tomorrow" to be an optional activity.

By the time restrictions eased, Chase had not only survived his trial-by-fire introduction to adulthood—he had *thrived*. Sure, he had some questionable budgeting habits (do you really need three different streaming subscriptions, son?), and I had to remind him more than once that cleaning wasn't just a *once-a-month* event, but overall? He did it.

He did it.

The day Chase moved out, part of me thought I would fall apart. I thought I would crumble under the weight of worry, imagining every possible scenario where he would need me and I wouldn't be there. Part of me was so excited that we had made this milestone! It was probably 80% worry and 10% excitement one day and the opposite the next.

But then, he proved that he could do it.

And I realised—he had been listening all along. Through the chaos, through the nagging, through the moments where I thought he wasn't paying attention—he had been absorbing some of what I had tried to teach him.

That was what mattered.

That was what I had been working towards all along.

But like all things challenges and hurdles get in the way of smooth sailing, and we have to adapt... again.

Chase vs. The Real World – A Comedy of Errors (and Tears)

Graduating high school is supposed to be this glorious moment where you throw your cap in the air and march bravely into the future. For Chase, it was more like tripping off the stage, landing face-first into adulthood, and realizing that no one was waiting with a safety net.

His post-high school life came with an unwelcome sidekick: depression. And I have to admit, I probably helped shove it into his life like an overenthusiastic matchmaker. I wanted so much for him, refused to acknowledge limitations, and pushed him harder than a malfunctioning shopping trolley. He was independent, living alone in his flat, but keeping a job? That was another story.

See, bosses love when employees show initiative. Chase... well, *does not have initiative*. Literally. His IQ sits at 70, and his cognitive abilities make everyday tasks feel like solving a Rubik's cube blindfolded. The world claims to be inclusive, but let's be honest—it has the patience of a toddler and the empathy of a rock.

Chase landed casual work, which meant zero job security, and when you have CF, *you get sick*. But rent doesn't care about your lungs, so he had to work. Hospital stays? Not an option—miss too many shifts, and he'd lose the flat. Coming home wasn't possible either; life had changed too much. So, every weekend, I'd show up, armed with cleaning supplies and groceries, scolding him for the bombsite I inevitably walked into. We pushed through together—sometimes hating each other, sometimes barely speaking—but we *did not quit*.

The big goal? Survive ten years in Australia so he could finally apply for government assistance. Until then, Chase was on his own financially. I had stubbornly believed he needed to work, that a benefit would trap him in poverty. But I had to let that nonsense go. Chase needed help. I couldn't do it all anymore. He was an adult, whether the world liked it or not.

For two and a half years, he fought to stay afloat. He had nine jobs. *Nine.* He gave them everything he had. It just wasn't enough.

Some bosses were kind but still had to let him go. Others were absolute nightmares. Like the one who asked, when Chase couldn't recite a scripted customer interaction word-for-word, whether he was a *"retard."* (Oh yes, that really happened. I had some *thoughts* about that one.) Or the boss who fired him for "underperformance," only to call him back a few hours later when they realised, they were short-staffed for six weeks. Chase said yes, of course. I wanted him to scream *no*, but money was money.

His confidence took a dive. He had gone from being school captain to being unable to hold down a job. He even lost a job washing cars. *Washing cars.* He was let go from cleaning a school because he wasn't *fast enough*. And when he dared to ask a boss what else he could do after finishing his assigned tasks, the man told him to *use his bloody initiative*—and fired him that Friday as he walked out the gate.

That day, Chase cried. He doesn't cry often. He's as tough as they come. But that one broke him. And it broke me too.

As if the job market wasn't savage enough, Chase also had to deal with a medical system that isn't exactly designed for adults with CF. Because let's be real—adults with CF aren't *supposed* to exist, right? This disease is meant to kill.

And yet... here we are.

Still fighting. Still standing. Still laughing at the absurdity of it all, because honestly, what else can you do?

The world might not be built for Chase, but neither was high school, neither was independence, and yet, he found his way. It's messy. It's frustrating. But it's *his* life. And despite everything, he's still living it.

And that folks is how we raised Chase!

As I wrap this story up, Chase is about to head to hospital for a two-week admission. He became an Australian Citizen two weeks ago opening up a previously restricted healthcare system. Despite having health insurance from the moment, we landed here in Australia all those years ago, Chase has been locked out of the additional support he needs to thrive. The system helped me keep him alive, but now it will help us work together so he can thrive.

We hope with support, he will be able to access services that will connect him to like-minded people, provide meal support and even social housing where he won't be so alone. There are weeks where he can go, and I am the only person he talks to. That is profoundly sad. That's not living – that is existing and like before something my vey being rallies against.

With support from the right people, he will be able to participate in life more fully while still maintaining his fragile health. He spent a few days at home recently where he and I worked on giving him a head start on this hospital admission.

I feel thankful that the people within the education and medical systems once they have spent time with Chase, real time not just a casual encounter, see the challenges he faces. The medical crisis his body has when he experiences DIOS. Now DIOS is a doozy!

Distal Intestinal Obstruction Syndrome (DIOS) is basically your intestines throwing a full-blown tantrum because they just can't deal. Imagine a traffic jam on the busiest highway in your gut—except instead of honking cars, it's thick, sticky mucus and stubborn poop refusing to move. This delightful disaster is a VIP experience for people with cystic fibrosis, thanks to their extra-sticky digestive juices turning their intestines into a slow-moving sludge factory. Symptoms range from "I just need to fart" discomfort to full-blown "Call an ambulance, my stomach is staging a rebellion." Treatment usually involves an unholy alliance of laxatives, fluids, and sometimes medical intervention to break up the blockage. It's like dealing with a plumbing emergency, except the pipes are your intestines, and the clog is way, way more personal.

And you don't find out about this until your kid starts vomiting poo... yep you read that right. It is gross extraordinarily weird and frankly out of this mum's comprehension range. But Chase would – back then we had no idea what it was. Now we do and we work to manage it. Chase's inability to grasp that if he chewed his food more, or ate more already broken-down food, balanced his meals, ate smaller meals more often instead of bingeing it might not happen as often. It continues to eventuate every six months or so and we just rinse and repeat. Metamucil to Chases disgust, and time at home where I manage his meals.

There are many medical issues that eventuate over time with CF. In the beginning it's the lungs... it gently merges into gut issues, then brittle bones and add CF-related diabetes (CFRD), where the pancreas, already slacking on its enzyme duties, decides to also mess up insulin production. Osteoporosis can sneak in too because malabsorption issues mean bones miss out on all the good stuff they need to stay strong. Liver disease might make an appearance, courtesy of bile ducts getting clogged with mucus like a bad plumbing job. Then there's chronic sinus infections, gastrointestinal disasters like DIOS and fertility challenges (especially in men, thanks to blocked or missing vas deferens). And let's not forget the mental health side—because juggling all these medical surprises while trying to adult like everyone else is, frankly, exhausting. CF keeps things... interesting, to say the least!

But at 23 years old on the precipice of something special, we celebrate each milestone.

He has travelled, met amazing people, conversed with a prime minister (and they still stay in touch!), has been a stepdad for a very short time of which we were incredibly proud of how he stepped up. It wasn't to work out long term, but that wee baby girl gave Chase the chance to experience pure love. He has faced incredible trials including a court case where he had to defend himself against serious but false accusations. He won. It left terrible scars on his soul.

He has learned that not all family relationships are perfect, but he has also discovered the strength in setting boundaries and valuing those who lift him up. He has faced the heartbreak of losing friends, grandparents, and beloved pets, yet through each loss, he has grown in resilience, cherishing the love and memories they left behind. Through it all, he has come to understand that while life brings challenges, it also offers deep connections, lessons in love, and the ability to keep moving forward with an open heart.

He is Chase.

And for you my reader, may you be blessed with deep rosy pink bellows of life that work without thought.

Donna

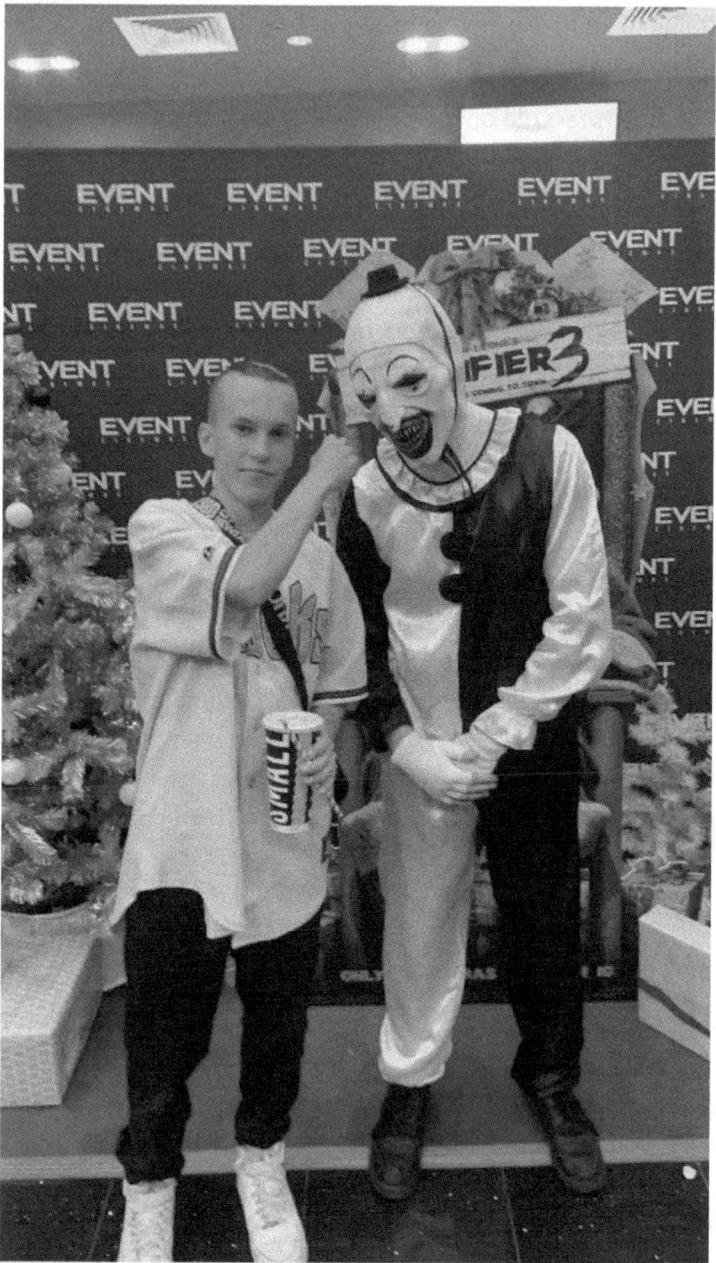

www.ingramcontent.com/pod-product-compliance
Lightning Source LLC
Chambersburg PA
CBHW061146040426
42445CB00013B/1571